Shane "The People's Chemist" Ellison, M.S.

D1096703

The 'Stop Eating So F#@%ing Much' Diet

Why Your Hormones Conspire Against You... and Why Diet Gurus are Full of Sh$t

The People's Chemist, LLC
2013

The 'Stop Eating So F#@%ing Much' Diet

Why Your Hormones Conspire Against You... and Why Diet Gurus are Full of Sh$t

By: The People's Chemist

For information contact:
support@thepeopleschemist.com
Publisher: The People's Chemist, LLC
Author: Shane "The People's Chemist" Ellison, M.S.
Web: www.thepeopleschemist.com

Disclaimer:
This is not medical advice. This book was written to help you look better naked. You may even use it to avoid Type II diabetes, heart disease and cancer. It will never be a cure for The Whine Flu. The reader agrees to take full responsibility for his or her own life decisions and understands that if they have The Whine Flu, the best cure is to first acknowledge it, then move forward.

Printed in Canada

"It doesn't take huge sacrifice to be fit and healthy, only hormones."

Table of Contents

Author's Note

The Internet is a great tool for getting the weather, downloading music, spying on friends via Facebook, and finding the latest deals on books, grass-fed beef and natural medicine. But, when it comes to learning how to achieve your best body, it can be a colossal waste of time, money and energy.

No matter where you click, an ad for the latest fad diet awaits. Adorned with cheesy sales-copy promising one-minute abs or pushing the latest fat melting wonder pills, slimming algae or some other diet craze, nobody is free from the diet guru propaganda.

There's the hCG Diet, Jenny Craig, Paleo, High-Protein and even more outlandish, the Morning Banana Diet. If you're looking to be a part of something more prestigious, you can always adhere to The Park Avenue Diet... or maybe something a bit more sexy like the South Beach Diet, where you can enjoy delicious, processed foods made with dozens of lab-derived, flavor mimics and artificial ingredients.

What? None of these worked?

Then perhaps you should try counting calories... or counting fat grams... or weighing every morsel of food on a kitchen scale... or take part in a new exercise fad... or become a vegetarian or vegan...

With so many conflicting ideas and billions of dollars in marketing thrown behind them, it's no wonder that so many people are confused about what it really takes to lose weight, be healthy and live young.

The answer is certainly not found in any of these unsustainable trends, which are designed for mass appeal, rather than safety and efficacy. That's why most "diets" fail their fans. They focus on sacrifice and denial short term and they actually work against your body long term! Dozens of controlled studies have shown only minimal weight loss with even the most popular diets. And for every "success story" the weight almost always comes back... and then some!

The New England Journal of Medicine published a two-year study of the weight loss efforts of more than 200 overweight people who followed many different diet plans. The average weight loss was about eight pounds – **after two years!**

So, if diets don't work, then maybe the solution is more "cardio."

Unfortunately, the conventional wisdom about cardiovascular fitness is just as flawed as it is about how and what we should eat. In fact, if you take part in long periods of "cardio" the way most diet gurus, government health agencies and medical organizations suggest, you will almost certainly GAIN weight and ruin your health!

Led by Joseph Proietto of the University of Melbourne's Department of Medicine, researchers showed that when the untrained body detects hunger from calorie deprivation and long bouts of exercise, a vast array of fat storing and appetite stimulating hormones spring to life. This survival mechanism helped pre-historic man–who had very few food choices–find the motivation and energy to hunt and supported life during unplanned periods of fasting. But today's diets leave modern man feeling hungry and heavy.

Diet gurus and most physicians never recognize this inherent flaw in dieting. Instead, they blame your brain, your mood, your emotions, or your genetics for abandoning their diet or exercise programs. They're full of shit.

When you deny your body of calories via dieting and simultaneously force it into a long "cardio" routine, your hormones eventually conspire against you by eliciting wanton food cravings. Eventually, whether its low-carb, no-carb, low-fat, organic, vegetarian, vegan, fruit and vegetables or eating like a club-carrying caveman, you're going to end up eating too fucking much! And you'll kill the hormones that regulate metabolism and longevity.

...That's what everyone's forgetting. It's all about hormones.

And that's why I wrote this book: to provide a step-by-step blueprint for rapidly restoring your healing hormones so you can enjoy your best body and health, at any age. Along the way, I'll dispel the dietary myths and lies that are keeping people fat and sick. But most importantly, I'll show you how to stop overeating forever and love life in the process.

The Key is to Work with Your Hormones, Not Against Them

Losing weight fast and keeping it off–while building lean sexy muscle, forever can be virtually effortless when you learn to work with your hormones. The permanent solution you're looking for has nothing to do with deprivation, denial or sacrifice.

That means you can say goodbye to never-ending workouts and "just say no" to bland boring food. And while you're at it, gather up all your "diet" books and throw them in the trash.

There is no "secret" to having the body you desire and the health you deserve.

It's all controlled by your hormones...

Hormones are everything. They determine how much you eat and when. Whether you burn fat... or store it. They determine whether you feel energetic and satisfied after a meal... or lethargic and prone to cravings. They determine whether you feel groggy and cranky in the mornings...or rested and rejuvenated.

Most importantly, your hormones determine whether you are traveling a path toward disease and early demise... or a lifetime of youthful activity and healthy longevity.

And the bottom line is that YOU control your hormones!

That is exactly what this book will help you accomplish. You are about to discover a wildly effective way to use food, exercise and nutritional supplements the right way using my "Hormone Intelligence Therapy," (HIT) to put a stop to unruly hormones that make you eat yourself into an early grave.

Where all previous attempts by modern medicine have focused on using hormone mimics, like thyroid medication or "bioidenticals," you'll be shown how to force your body–or more specifically your DNA–to better utilize its own internal pharmacy to control appetite and optimize lean body mass, energy, libido, mood, willpower and all the other things the diet gurus blamed you for not having, yet were the result of their flimsy protocols and ill-thought out dietary advice.

This is not a boring thesis on appetite control or the biological mechanisms of obesity, insulin resistance and diabetes. The science jargon has been kept to a minimum.

This is a call to action – a step-by-step plan to lose 2–3 pounds of fat each week until you obtain your "best body" with minimal effort and no suffering.

For the first time in history, there are more obese people than their are thin ones. And our lifespan is dwindling because of it. Follow this plan and you'll rapidly become a **HIT Man** or **HIT Woman** – someone who has reached their full genetic potential, courtesy of proper hormone output, balance and sensitivity–and you won't be a part of the new majority. Hormone intelligence will manifest into vibrant health and longevity as well as your optimal physique in the shortest time possible!

Dare to live young,

Shane Ellison, MS
The People's Chemist
www.thepeopleschemist.com

Introduction

The Hormone Intelligence Therapy Breakthrough

We are currently experiencing the most widespread disease and obesity epidemic the world has ever known.

As I am writing to you today, two out of three Americans are overweight. Diabetes is nine times more likely than it was just 30 years ago. Heart disease kills over a million people each year in the U.S. alone. And as the "Standard American Diet" (SAD) is exported worldwide, the problems of obesity and chronic disease go with it.

If you are struggling with your weight and your health, then this book is for you. On the other hand, if you're fortunate enough to be in reasonably good health and have avoided obesity, don't be fooled into thinking you have nothing to worry about... or that 30, 20 or even 10 pounds of flab won't hurt you.

In fact, the health consequences of being even slightly overweight can be substantial. According to the *North American Association for the Study of*

Obesity, gaining just 20 pounds in adulthood DOUBLES your risk of diabetes and more than doubles your risk of hypertension!

The leaner you are, the better you will look, the better you will feel, and the longer you will be able to enjoy your health.

The great news is that your body is pre-programmed for optimal health. You are designed to be lean and strong. And you are built to be active, well into your later years.

The problem for most of us is that the habits we have fallen into – what we eat and how we exercise (or don't exercise) – have radically disrupted our hormonal systems. As a result, we are suffering from what I call, "hormonal ignorance."

What is Hormonal Ignorance?

The modern day plague of hormonal ignorance is marked by three biological shortcomings:

1. Poor Hormone Output

2. Poor Hormone Balance

3. Poor Hormone Sensitivity

At first, victims of hormonal ignorance experience poor energy, depression, and a lack of sexual potency and desire. Over time, it can even change your physical appearance, resulting in accelerated aging, wrinkles and poor complexion. Ultimately, the most serious long-term manifestations of hormonal ignorance are Type II diabetes, heart disease, cancer and almost every other chronic disease known to man.

And of course, hormonal ignorance can also earn you a guaranteed place in the "Fat Cow Hall of Fame," as it did me...

When your body is hormonally ignorant your appetite rages, causing you to keep eating when you should feel satisfied. You face undeniable cravings, despite your best efforts to ignore them. Your body also becomes programmed to store fat instead of burning it.

As the years go by, the weight continues to accumulate and losing it becomes virtually impossible.

When hormonal ignorance reigns, a total lack of harmony sets in. Life-sustaining testosterone, estrogen, thyroid hormones, human growth hormone (hGH), leptin, ghrelin, amylin, cholescystokinin, glucagon, insulin and so many others cease to function properly.

There is no drug that will save you from the modern affliction of hormonal ignorance. Not even the highly touted Bioidentical Hormone Replacement Therapy (BHRT) can increase your body's own hormone output. Nor can they restore your hormone balance or "re-sensitize" you to your "God-given hormones" that restore health and youthful vigor.

But that doesn't mean there is no solution, because...

You Can Control Your Hormone State

Just like winds direct the movement of clouds, hormones direct biological actions in your body. They are messenger molecules that send a myriad of bio-chemical signals, which control and stimulate a fleet of enzymes, neurotransmitters and other compounds.

Your hormones help to orchestrate your breathing rate, heartbeat, oxygen delivery, cellular water balance, caloric intake and even your emotions. They can also turn on life-enhancing genes while turning the deadly ones off. And they also play a huge role when it comes to your body composition.

Your hormones help regulate your metabolism, they stimulate or relieve your hunger, they regulate your blood sugar... and they control whether you store fat or burn it, and build muscle.

When your body has "hormone intelligence," it means that you are *producing* **just the right amounts of each hormone and that these hormones are** *perfectly balanced* **in relation to one another. It also means that your body is** *highly sensitive* **to the effects of the hormones you produce.**

This is an incredibly delicate and complex process, but it's surprisingly easy to control. And you don't have to know anything about how it works. But, you do need to know that hormone intelligence is your body's natural state of balance and equilibrium. That means you will innately gravitate toward this set point, if you just get out of the way and start working with your body, instead of against it.

The "intelligence" that plants use to capture sunlight or take up nutrients from the soil and convert these things into energy for growth is the same intelligence your body uses to heal itself naturally and preserve a healthy physique. It is perfectly natural and happens without you even having to think about it.

The key is to master a few critical hormones like insulin, glucagon, estrogen and testosterone through my Hormone Intelligence Therapy (HIT) program, outlined in this book. Once you control these key hormones as a HIT Man or HIT Woman, your entire hormonal chain of command – like an orchestra playing in perfect unison – will be in your hands.

You will be able to harness your own internal pharmacy to produce weapons of fat destruction and optimal genetic expression!

By re-programming your hormonal chemistry, you can easily transform your body into a perpetual fat-burning, muscle building machine and reclaim your youthful fitness and vitality.

The Changes You Seek Can Happen Faster than You Imagine

It doesn't matter how old or out of shape you might be at the moment. You can still have the body you used to have… or the body you always wished you had. And the changes can begin within days!

Based on my own results and those of thousands of clients over the years, here's just part of what you are going to accomplish as you follow the **Hormone Intelligence Therapy Breakthrough**:

- Lean, sexy muscle will begin to emerge as your body begins to melt fat and turn it into energy

- Your blood pressure and resting heart rate will move toward optimal levels, while your heart and lungs will grow more powerful

- Any puffiness in your face will begin to disappear, your skin and eyes will glow and your complexion will improve

- Your risk of diabetes, heart disease and cancer will be reduced substantially

- Your immune system will become stronger and more resistant

- You will feel less stress and anxiety and a greater sense of energy and well-being

- Your sleep will improve and you will notice greater physical and mental energy

- Your appetite will be more balanced and between-meal cravings will disappear

- Prostate health will be at its best

- You will stop being plagued by cravings

- You will notice greater sexual desire and potency... and much more!

- You will stop eating so fucking much... and much more!

But before we get started, it's important that you know what qualifies me to lead you down this path. It's not because I read these ideas in books or even the medical literature. Although there are hundreds of studies which support these principles and I have used many of them to create this program.

The real foundation for what you are about to learn comes from my direct personal experience and nearly a dozen years of working with clients and customers just like you.

Chapter 1: Eight Weight Loss Lies that Can Permanently Harm You

I confess… I used to be "overweight."

Scratch that… I was fat. But it didn't start out like that. As a wrestler in college, I clocked in at a lean and mean 4% body fat. That's about the level of an elite bodybuilder.

But as time passed into my late 20s, I ballooned to a whopping 30% body fat.

I felt weak and tired and I was constantly haunted by cravings for food — usually anything that tasted sweet. These cravings ate at me from the inside and would overcome even my staunchest efforts at willpower. They came on as fast as the Oatmeal Pies went down.

I would even have cravings right after a big meal. I was eating and drinking more than enough calories. Yet, I was still "hungry" – or so I thought.

My mood and energy levels would also swing wildly. I was often edgy and depressed. And I always felt like I needed a nap about two o'clock in the afternoon. But there was one thing that always seemed to boost my mood and energy (at least for a little while) – more carbs!

As my belt size continued to grow, it became more and more strenuous just to follow a basic exercise routine. Slowly but surely, my body felt like it was shutting down.

As I became disgusted by my own body and tired of the way I felt, I grew determined to awaken from my metabolic nightmare and lose the unwanted fat, while building muscle in the shortest time possible.

I didn't want to be the guy who had poor libido and no strength. I didn't want to be the fat guy at the beach anymore. And I sure as hell didn't want to be the sad-sack sifting through a drawer full of orange pill bottles at sunrise looking for my blood pressure medications and cholesterol-lowering drugs, while the healthy guys were gallivanting at the gym or strutting around the block for their morning run!

But I have to admit, that as an organic chemist trained in biochemistry and drug design, my first instinct was to look to pills as a potential cure for my ever-expanding belly. Don't forget, this was when I was still employed by the pharmaceutical industry and just beginning my study of natural medicine.

I mapped out the actions of each and every drug that was purported to aid in weight loss – including Wellbutrin, Phentermine, Xenical, Clenbuterol, Meridia and amphetamines. Not a single one had a study to prove they could rid me of my excess fat. But plenty of research highlighted their risks.

I also researched thyroid medications like Synthroid and Armour Thyroid, which are hyped with promises of a thinner waist and enhanced hormone balance. But, these drugs proved to be nothing more than a clever scam targeting women, because weight control and metabolism are only slightly managed by the thyroid. This is evidenced by those who have had their thyroid surgically removed but remain slim, as well as by those who take thyroid meds but fail to lose weight.

Finally, I studied volumes of research available on various fad diets, strenuous exercise programs, and the recommendations of various health agencies, including the government mandated "Food Pyramid."

I didn't want to be the yo-yo on a new yo-yo diet every six months or the one carrying around a dorky food and exercise journal. But I was willing to try just about anything to regain the fitness and strength of my youth.

As time went by, I tried several of these programs, including a few "fad" diets. Not surprisingly, I always ended up in the same place: mediocre results that were temporary at best. Most were a complete waste of time and money, not to mention a drain on my health.

Eventually, I went back to my roots as a chemist and discovered what I believe is the Holy Grail of fitness and health – hormone intelligence. In just a moment, I'll tell you everything you need to know about it and just how easy it is to achieve your best body and vibrant health.

But first, it's critical that you understand the lies and myths that are out there about weight loss and exercise. If you follow these flawed theories, it could seriously undermine your health... not to mention make your fat loss efforts virtually impossible to maintain.

Weight Loss Lie #1:
The hCG Diet is Safe and Effective

I could write an entire book debunking the most popular fad diets with proven science and real results. Most of these diets either promote fake foods with artificial ingredients, they are focused on counting this or cutting out that, or they are simply based on erroneous and unscientific conclusions.

The bottom line is that very few of these diets will produce any results at all, much less, results that are lasting and significant. So, I won't be saying much more about fad diets in this book. But there is one that I do want to address, due to its recent popularity. I'm talking about the hCG Diet.

The hCG Diet was actually devised by a physician in 1954. And despite the fact that the hypothesis was disproven many years ago, it has reemerged, thanks to the Chicago-based marketing whiz and bestselling author, Kevin Trudeau. Many have heard of it, but few understand it. So I'm going to sum it up: It's another fad diet destined to steal the hopes and dreams of fat people everywhere. Here are a few telling quotes I pulled from online message forums:

"I used hCG in my bodybuilding years. It ruined my metabolism and made me fatter years later..." – Sandi

"I'm worried about my wife. She started the hCG diet and is looking weak, pale and is very lethargic." – Dan

Weight loss often does plummet when the diet begins. But this is due to the severe restriction in calories, causing the body to lose glycogen and muscle, while holding fat. Many users incorrectly identify this as a measure of success, simply based on a lower number on the scale. But hCG has never been proven to cause healthy fat loss while preserving life-sustaining muscle.

And that's the least of the bad news…

The really bad news is that, over the long run, the hCG diet can lead to overt obesity, as well as type II diabetes and even cancer! Before you let the Trudeau marketing noose tighten around your neck, here are a few things you must know about the hCG diet.

The first hormone produced by a pregnant woman is hCG. It primes her body for carrying the new baby. In particular, it turns on the flow of progesterone and estrogen. These are the "Honey, I think I'm gaining weight, can you buy me a pregnancy test," hormones! If not controlled, the estrogen dominance may lead to weight gain at first, then type II diabetes.

The hCG diet hucksters try to mask this symptom by telling users to go on a "very low calorie diet." But, since starvation isn't sustainable, the yo-yo effect kicks in faster than you can say "Natural Cures I Wish I Didn't Know About."

But the hCG hormone isn't a one-trick pony. In addition to turning on the flow of progesterone and estrogen, it also preserves the early stages of pregnancy. However, for those not pregnant, hCG preserves cancer growth by acting as a life-support for this biological superpower.

Specifically, hCG grants cancerous cells the ability to produce blood vessels, a process known technically as neovascularization. *The scientific journal, Anticancer Research*, highlighted this in 2003, stating that, "hCG is able to induce neovascularization in tumor cells."

The hCG Diet does not produce sustainable weight loss, nor is it safe. Helping cancer cells to grow is not a good thing. Avoid the hCG diet.

Weight Loss Lie #2:
Low Fat Diets are the Key to Weight Loss & Health

If you want to lose fat, eating less of it seems to make a lot of sense. But that doesn't mean it's true.

The "low-fat" diet craze is more than 20 years old. And all we have to show for it is a population that is fatter and unhealthier than ever before. When manufacturers remove the fat from foods, they have to replace it with something. And more often than not, that "something" is sugar, so most "low-fat" and "fat-free" foods are high in refined carbohydrates.

But that's not the only problem with a low fat diet.

The word "fat" describes molecules that are made of long chains of carbon atoms, each with a characteristic acid group at the end. Most people simply know these compounds to be a high calorie food that they're supposed to avoid, thanks to USDA propaganda. But, for the most part, that propaganda is wrong and misleading.

The key is not to avoid fat. The key is to distinguish between healthy fats and unhealthy fats. You have to be selective about the fat you're boycotting, otherwise you risk hijacking your health.

The fats you want to AVOID are **trans fats** (look for the word "hydrogenated" on nutrition labels) and **omega-6 fats** (primarily from vegetable and seed oils). These harmful fats are primarily found in fast food and commercial fried foods, margarine products, "butter" sprays and spreads, salad dressings, chips, and just about every processed food on the market.

The slight molecular variation in these man-made and chemically-processed fats can cause serious health complications. As these biological impostors are incorporated into the gelatinous membranes of the cells, these membranes go from squishy and pliable to dry and brittle, causing cell function to deteriorate. Studies clearly show that these two types of fat promote inflammation and obesity and increase your risk of diabetes, cancer, heart disease and more.

And if you look around you, this is the path that most Americans are following. But the same is not true for naturally-occurring fats found in grass-fed beef and butter, pastured pork and poultry, fish, eggs, nuts, avocados, olives and coconuts. In fact, the **saturated fats, monounsaturated fats and omega-3 fats** found in these foods actually promote health and protect against disease.

Instead of promoting inflammation, these healthy fats quell it. Instead of adding to the flab on your belly, butt and thighs and surrounding your organs, these fats actually help you burn it. And rather than causing cells to become dry and brittle, these fats help to form the squishy, gelatinous membranes that ensure proper cell function and preserve a youthful complexion.

Finally, healthy fats also help to carry vital micronutrients throughout your body. When you consume a very low fat diet, many of these vital "fat soluble" nutrients are eliminated without even being digested.

Foods that contain healthy fats should be the mainstay of your diet. Not only will these foods help to satisfy your hunger for hours, they also won't spike your blood sugar. In fact, because many hormones – especially testosterone – are produced in fat cells, consuming healthy fat is vital if you wish to achieve hormone intelligence.

The bottom line is that the right dietary fats are not only beneficial, they are absolutely essential for shedding fat and improving your body composition.

Weight loss may occur on a low-fat diet, but you will sacrifice your health and appearance, as you lose muscle, cell function drops, energy plummets, and your skin begins to sag and wrinkle. Low fat diets are not safe or effective.

Weight Loss Lie #3:
Exercise is the Key to Fat Loss

Over the last 28 years, I've taken part in all types of fitness in pursuit of the endorphin high – swimming, weight lifting, wrestling, adventure racing and mountain biking, to name a few. During this same time, I've been fit enough to be mistaken for the "Man Your Man Could Smell Like" from the Old Spice commercials (just kidding) and fat enough to be an honorary member of The Fat Cow Hall of Fame (not kidding).

But regardless of the amount of physical exertion I put forth, my body weight still yo-yo'd out of control. I quickly learned that exercising as a method for burning calories is not nearly as important as what you put in your mouth.
You might have heard the saying that, "You can't out-train a bad diet." That's because it can take only minutes to consume far more calories than you could burn even during two hours of intense exercise.

For example, a few slices of pizza and a tall glass of Coke, would set you back about 1,000 calories. A McDonald's Big Mac, large soft drink and large fries: 1,624 calories. A Starbucks Mocha Frappucino: 450 calories.

Now consider what it takes to burn off the energy you consume. The table (Table 1) below shows how many calories a 130 pound person and a 180 pound person would burn, while engaged in various physical activities.

As you can see, the average man would have to run or play full court basketball for almost two hours just to burn off three slices of pizza and a soft drink. The average woman would have to run for almost THREE HOURS to burn off the same meal.

When you consider these facts, it's crystal clear that exercise is NOT the most important part of the fat loss equation. And that's not even the worst of it, because if you work out the way most exercise gurus and health agencies recommend, you will almost certainly GAIN weight!

The typical recommendation from mainstream health organizations is to engage in long-duration cardio. While "cardio" exercise does burn calories, long workouts will also make you ravenously hungry. And numerous studies have shown that people who exercise more tend to eat more. And as we have just seen, it is a lot easier to consume those calories than it is to burn them!

Finally, long duration endurance exercise also causes your levels of human growth hormone and testosterone to fall... while causing levels of cortisol (a stress hormone) to rise. This is the definition of hormonal ignorance, and virtually guarantees the loss of muscle and the accumulation of fat. For evidence, just take a look at the flat chests, flabby arms, and skinny legs of most marathon runners.

To make exercise count, you must be hormonally intelligent. Just like a hybrid car is able to use different sources of energy, your body can use different types of fuel for work. And it is your hormones that dictate what type of fuel that will be. When you are hormonally ignorant, your body will burn sugar and break down protein for energy, while holding on to fat at all costs.

However, as a HIT Man or HIT Woman, your body will be programmed to burn fat as its preferred source of energy, and it will do so around the clock.

Table 1: Calories Burned Per Hour of Exercise

Activity	130 lbs.	180 lbs.
Jiu Jitsu / Wrestling	590	817
Full court basketball	472	690
Running (12 minute mile)	472	690
Stationary Bicycle (moderate)	413	604
Golf, carrying clubs	325	474
Walking (brisk pace)	224	311

Exercise is definitely part of the fat-loss equation, but the foods you eat and your ability to control your hormones are far more important than how much time you sweat in the gym.

Weight Loss Lie #4:
The Food Pyramid is the Ideal Food Guide

The U.S. Department of Health and the USDA recommend that a healthy diet should consist of 6–11 servings of bread, cereal, rice and pasta... DAILY! This has become the basis of our national nutrition policy and the party line for government licensed "registered dieticians."

Hopefully, I don't have to tell you that this is the perfect recipe for obesity and poor health. But you might wonder, where did these misguided recommendations come from? They certainly didn't come from the halls of science.

The idea that the foundation of a healthy diet should come from grains is largely the result of the Food Guide Pyramid, devised through a joint endeavor by the U.S. Department of Health and Human Services and the USDA in 1992.

As it was originally designed, The Food Pyramid would have been a benefit to public health. Luise Light, MS, Ed.D., the scientist who led the team which created the original Food Pyramid, stated that the original plan recommended very minimal grains, along with a balanced array of healthy fats, proteins and carbohydrates from fruits and vegetables.

But the Food Pyramid that was designed by Light and her team was very different from the one that was eventually released to the public. At the request of the processed food industry, crackers, cereal, bread, pasta and baked goods were moved to the base of the pyramid, where they were to make up the bulk of the American diet.

Of course, these changes had nothing to do with improving nutrition – and everything to do with improving the profits of the food industry!

The Food Pyramid has recently been changed to a new infographic, referred to as My Plate, which was designed by a PR firm that also represents McDonald's and the Snack Food Association. Not surprisingly, while the design has changed, the recommendations are still the same.

My Plate ignores nutrient-rich, naturally-occurring proteins and fats, while recommending that at least 50% of your diet consist of whole grains – things like amaranth, barley, buckwheat, corn, millet, oats, rice, rye, sorghum, teff and wheat (including varieties such as spelt, emmer, einkorn, Kamut®, durum and forms such as bulgur and wheatberries).

You're better off eating Dog Chow than these foods, because it would keep your metabolism moving at a much higher rate.

Your body processes breads, cereals and starchy foods just like sugar. As your blood sugar rises, the pancreas produces a hormone "sugar taxi," known as insulin. This carries sugar out of the bloodstream and into the cells where it can be used for energy. **What you must remember is that the body will always burn sugar (if it is present) before burning fat. Therefore insulin and fat burning cannot co-exist.**

So every time you shove grains into your pie-hole, you're suffocating your fat-burning metabolism and causing your gut to get bigger.

Over time, excess sugar and insulin will cause muscle cells to become resistant to insulin, just like excess drinking leads to alcohol resistance. This causes cravings, lack of energy and, eventually, obesity, Type 2 diabetes and inflammation leading to heart disease and cancer... things that your neighbors suffer from.

Without a doubt, The Food Pyramid and My Plate are not the ideal food guides. They are nothing more than a thinly disguised marketing scheme for major food companies like Kellogg's and General Mills to push their packaged, processed, high-profit margin, whole-grain foods.

Anyone who adheres to the nutritional and dietary guidelines set by the Department of Health and the USDA will eventually become an honorary member of The Fat Cow Hall of Fame.

Weight Loss Lie #5:
Calorie Restriction is an Effective
Weight Loss Strategy

Before I dispel this pervasive myth, it's important to note that if your goal is to lose weight and improve your body composition, you MUST maintain a calorie deficit. That means you have to burn more calories than you consume.

But that does not mean that you need to count calories and it certainly doesn't mean starving yourself. Effective and permanent fat loss is not about deprivation and denial or having the willpower to overcome nagging hunger for days on end.

In fact, as long as you follow the recommendations in this book, you should rarely be hungry at all (and never ravenously). The key is to eat satiating food, like healthy fats and protein, which will keep you full for hours. It's also about mastering your hormones, so your appetite is regulated and your cravings disappear.

I'll show you how to do that momentarily. But for now, let's discuss why you should never "starve" yourself to lose weight.

One of the greatest perils our ancestors faced was a shortage of food. To overcome the threat of famine, we adapted the ability to slow down our metabolism. After all, the more "mileage" you get from the energy you consume, the longer you can endure without food.

There is no doubt that if you have the willpower, you can lose weight by starving yourself. The problem is that your body doesn't know the difference between a "diet" and a famine. In response to a significant and prolonged reduction in calories, your metabolism will slow down and your hormones will send the signal to store fat, instead of burning it.

And that's not all. Studies also show that anywhere from 20% – 40% of the weight lost on very low calorie diets is the result of muscle loss.

For most of us, there is no way to sustain such deprivation for the long term. Eventually, you will start eating normally again. And when you do, your lethargic metabolism will continue to burn fewer calories and your hormones will ensure that those calories are stored as fat. And while the fat will return faster than ever, the muscle may never return at all.

If you want to maximize fat loss, you need to boost your metabolism, not slow it down.

Weight Loss Lie #6:
Small Meals throughout the day
Spark Your Metabolism

Here is another way to get fat long term: Feed your face 4–6 times daily (also known as grazing).

The first things I think of when I hear the term "grazing" are fat farm animals. But this image has failed to deter fit hopefuls. The grazing myth grew from the discovery that eating boosts your metabolism. It's called diet-induced thermogenesis (DIT). I learned about it in 9th grade, along with all the other outdated, simple-minded personal training drab found in muscle magazines.

But there is a limit to everything. And the limit to diet induced thermogenesis diminishes after three meals. Otherwise, why not eat 10 meals a day? Duh. My 5-year old calls it "eating too often."

With respect to controlling weight, an excessive number of meals only works for people who are severely restricting calories, addicted to exercise, or injecting steroids like a 'roided out bodybuilder. These three actions counter the fat-inflating side effects of "eating too much" by forcing the body to compensate with starvation, energy output, or hormones, respectively.

But anyone else adhering to the multi-meal myth is doomed, as proven by post-meal blood tests, DNA studies and the real-life outcomes of weight gain over time.

After a week or two of grazing, the body adapts to meal overload by pumping out the fat storing hormone insulin and simultaneously lowering fat crushing hormones like glucagon, testosterone and human growth hormone (hGH). This is a metabolic nightmare for people who dream about looking good naked.

When my wife Lea-Ann started a career in figure competitions, she dabbled in the four-to-six-meals-a-day dogma. She also suffered from weight gain rebound, or what her fitness competition cronies refer to as "post-competition bloat." She eventually came around.

In contrast, studies on low meal frequency, where food intake is restricted to every five hours, show the exact opposite results of multi-meal intake – low insulin and high amounts of the fat-crushing hormones glucagon, testosterone and hGH. The five hour window, considered short term fasting, forces the body to rid itself of food-induced insulin response, and then produce fat burning, muscle building hormones between meals.

Smaller, frequent meals disrupt this anti-aging process. The benefits of three meals per day can be verified in the real world with positive changes in lean body mass and increased athletic performance.

Applying low meal frequency to her training and supplement protocol, my wife experienced the benefits by winning the Arnold Amateur in 2009, without the post-competition rebound. By sticking to the easy-to-follow-protocol, she carries the same great physique today, with little sacrifice.

To verify the negative outcomes of the multi-meal myth first hand, attend a bodybuilding event where the belief runs deep. Pay attention to the ex-participants. Scurrying around in tight shirts and pants that won't let go of their thighs, they're traditionally overweight, especially in the gut and chest, where multi-meal insulin overload "weighs heavy," giving rise to the spare tire hanging off the waist and "moobs," slung low from the chest, now popularized by famed 'roider and bodybuilder Arnold Schwarzenegger.

The cultural dogma among the bodybuilding community and its long term side-effect of obesity and accelerated aging is a poignant reminder that muscles and health don't always go hand in hand, and that small meals throughout the day don't spark metabolism.

Weight Loss Lie #7:
Low Carb Diets are the Best Diets

There are many variations of the low-carb diet. While some gurus advocate higher amounts of healthy fat in place of carbohydrates, others push for higher protein. In general, the higher-healthy-fat approach to the low-carb diet can be ideal for people who suffer from a metabolic illness such as obesity, insulin resistance, and Type II diabetes.

Still, neither of these diets are optimal, because healthy individuals, and especially athletes, would face more risk than benefit when lowering carbohydrate intake to less than 50% of calories (as long as they choose the right carbs!). The best source of carbohydrates are non-sweet, naturally occurring complex carbohydrates found in vegetables.

The low-carb diet began in 1797, courtesy of Dr. John Rollo, who treated his diabetic patients by removing carbohydrates from their meals. The medical community followed his lead, and today most people are familiar with the diet as a result of the late Dr. Atkins, who advocated replacing carbohydrates with fats and a bit of protein for his obese, Type II diabetic patients.

More recently, the low-carb craze has been purported to lend a "metabolic advantage" to those who overeat, while pursuing a low-carb and high protein diet. But it's baloney. Overeating will always cause an energy imbalance that favors fat storage. Overeating is overeating, whether you are eating seeds, nuts or cotton candy. Although the hormonal effects will be different, the end result will still be weight gain.

Carbohydrates are **macronutrients** that come from foods like grains, dairy products, fruits, vegetables and legumes (beans and peas). Biochemically, they're known as saccharides, or molecular chains of sugar. Once consumed, your body breaks these chains into individual sugar units and your blood sugar rises to various degrees depending on the type and amount of carbohydrate you consumed.

To shuttle these sugary molecules out of your bloodstream, your pancreas produces insulin, which triggers the muscle cells to vacuum them up and use it as energy. For athletes and healthy individuals, this is a very efficient process. Sugar and insulin are rapidly taken up by the muscles.

But the opposite is true for those who are overweight and obese, Type II diabetics and individuals who frequently consume large amounts of carbohydrates. For these people, insulin and sugar linger in the bloodstream for long periods of time. This causes numerous health problems and ensures that your body's fat-burning furnace will stay permanently switched off!

Biochemists have also shown that excess insulin pushes testosterone, glucagon and other fat burning compounds out of the blood, causing overt weight gain and critical imbalances of these essential hormones.

Removing carbohydrates, helps the obese or Type II diabetic reverse the illness. By lowering (not eliminating) carbohydrate intake and replacing it with healthy fats (not just any fats), diabetics and the obese can rapidly change their metabolism from constantly burning sugar to burning fat instead.

At the cellular level this process gives rise to compounds called ketones, the byproducts of burning body fat at the most basic level – in the powerhouse of each cell, called the mitochondria. The more **ketones** that get charred through the cellular engine the better. Eventually, the low carb diet became the ketogenic diet.

However, if you're not insulin resistant, Type II diabetic, obese, or epileptic, the low carb diet can potentially cause serious problems. Excessively lowering carbohydrates removes an important source of micronutrients. But it also causes a weighty compound known as glycogen to quickly become depleted. Glycogen comprises about 8% of the human body mass and provides long term energy to the muscles, organs and brain cells. This is the first source of energy to be lost to a low-carb diet. The resulting weight loss is mistakenly thought of as a good thing among devoted followers of a ketogenic diet.

For fit people, the loss of glycogen and micronutrients from an excessive low-carb diet leads to muscle weakness, fatigue, poor thyroid function and the inability to think as clearly. Even worse, it can almost immediately cause irritability, aggravation and a short temper – a condition I call "psychoglycemia."

Brain cells use twice as much energy as all other cells in the body. And your brain cells cannot use fats and proteins to produce the fuel they need. The energy for the brain comes strictly from glycogen. And just as muscle cells can't function without water, brain cells are unable to produce enzymes and neurotransmitters that aid in memory and problem solving when glycogen and micronutrients plummet.

So, while low carb diets can be an effective therapeutic tool for the obese, Type II diabetics and epileptics, they are not applicable to the masses or those that are already healthy and fit. Among this population, the insulin rebound is fast. Therefore, they will not be metabolically shackled by healthy carb intake – even at 50%.

Weight Loss Lie #8:
Bioidentical Hormones Kick Start Metabolism as You Age

Bioidentical hormones can be very beneficial for women who have had hysterectomies. They have provided huge relief to those who would have otherwise been forced to risk the more dangerous Hormone Replacement Therapy (HRT). When used by this select population, under the careful guidance of a health professional who uses blood tests to gauge and monitor their safety and effectiveness, bioidentical hormones can provide a quality of life that would not be available, otherwise.

But for others, it's a shot in the dark. That's because "bioidenticals" are not really bioidentical, and over time, they can desensitize our body from its own hormones, causing long term consequences.

The term "bioidentical" is used to describe lab-created hormones known as estradiol, estrone, estriol (sometimes simply referred to as "estrogen"), progesterone, testosterone and dehydroepiandrosterone (DHEA). While they are similar to our own hormones and share the same name, they are NOT "identical" as has been claimed. The atoms that make up their structure – like the bricks of a home – are different than the atoms used by the body to produce them. Unknown to most patients, this important distinction is now well understood and has officially become a part of college chemistry text books.

In a recent statement, The International Union for Pure and Applied Chemistry underscores the difference between biological hormones produced by the body and bioidentical hormones, which are commonly used by athletes to gain a competitive edge:

"For the first time in history, a change will be made to the atomic weights found in the inside covers of chemistry text-books worldwide. In sports doping investigations, performance enhancing testosterone considered bioidentical can be identified in the human body because the atomic weight of natural human testosterone is higher than that of pharmaceutical testosterone."

This seemingly small molecular difference between "bioidenticals" and those produced by the body can make for big side effects. But hormone patients and athletes are unaware. Via the marketing ploys of "kick starting your metabolism" and "slowing down the hands of time," the use of bioidentical hormones has spread widely into the aging and obese populations who show low hormone production.

Admittedly, many users of bioidentical hormones report increased energy and alertness. But outside of their use for women who have had a hysterectomy, those who swear by the benefits of these chemicals are little different from a bodybuilder who swears by the use of steroids. Like many drug cocktails, bioidenticals can make people feel good. But their benefits can be short term and there are risks.

Unlike biologically produced hormones, bioidenticals not only desensitize our hormone receptors, they also bypass full processing in the liver. This causes the counterfeits to slowly build up, or bioaccumulate, in the body. As saturation continues, every "small" dose becomes a larger one in time and our tissues become overwhelmed. This alters our internal hormone landscape.

Like the wrong key being jammed into a lock, the body becomes severed from its natural hormonal output, balance and sensitivity. A slew of dangerous outcomes are possible, as shown by studies on the use of bioidentical estrogen, progesterone, and testosterone.

Estrogen can Increase Thyroid Cancer

Estrogen is made by men and women. However, it is the relative balance between this and other hormones that dictates its powerful effects on sexuality. Among a kaleidoscope of functions, estrogen directs thyroid function by binding to the gland and stimulating activity in much the same way that combustion in a car engine elicits wheel movement.

Too much estrogen puts thyroid cells into overdrive and raises the risk of cancer by igniting uncontrolled cell growth. Scientists writing for *the Journal of Thyroid Research* wrote that, "Carcinomas of the thyroid are three-times more frequent in women than in men, and the peak rates occur earlier in women. These epidemiological data suggest a role of estrogen in the pathogenesis of thyroid diseases."

Adding to the risk, uterine cancer is also cropping up among those with high estrogen. Over time, the accumulation causes thickening of the uterine wall, which strips cells of their innate ability to slough off and make way for new ones. As the aging uterine cells stack up, they begin to decay, yet continually replicate, giving rise to uncontrolled growth – cancer. To offset the cancer risk, many physicians prescribe bioidentical progesterone, which brings yet more risk!

Excess Progesterone can Lead to Stubborn Fat Growth

Bioidentical progesterone is a popular drug among menopausal women who are diagnosed with estrogen dominance – either as a result of increased estrogen levels or low progesterone output. But women who opt for the progesterone supplement face an increased risk of fat gain, muscle wasting and other risks over time.

Progesterone is primarily a pregnancy hormone. During the third trimester, levels are at their peak. In fact, progesterone can be 10 to 50 times higher at this time than it would be for the average non-pregnant woman (50–200 ng/ml versus 1–28 ng/ml on average). This is conducive to pregnancy because it forces the body to carry more fat calories (energy) for baby and mom.

The mechanism by which progesterone shifts a mom's metabolism to favor pregnancy is fascinating, because it highlights nature's innate ability to accommodate the birthing process and also serves as warning to potential bioidentical users. Like a blanket of smog over a city, progesterone covers insulin receptors – causing "insulin resistance." This happens as a means of activating energy storage, in the form of weight gain, and is later used for development and birthing.

Once mom has the baby, progesterone levels plummet and the insulin resistance is cured. (Assuming mom follows proper lifestyle habits.) Bioidentical patients aren't that lucky.

Artificial progesterone "bioaccumulates." That means the longer patients take it, the more they have in the body. Even the smallest doses can become very large ones over time. And just like in pregnancy, the excess progesterone fills the bloodstream, covers insulin receptors, and causes the pre-diabetic symptoms of severe weight gain and all the complications that come from it (including depression, lack of energy and an increased risk for heart disease and cancer).

Testosterone Can Feminize Men
Aging men – athletes too – will sometimes supplement with testosterone to counteract a reduced libido and declining muscle strength as their naturally produced levels of this hormone decline. Like a good wine buzz, bioidentical testosterone feels great at first. Combined with excess exercise and a rigid, low sugar/carbohydrate diet, its use can have profound effects on metabolism and male physique. The problems from testosterone use arise over time.

Today's bioidentical testosterone can become tomorrow's estrogen, thanks to a feminizing enzyme known as aromatase, which latches on to bioidentical testosterone molecules and converts them into estrogen! That's right, "bioidentical" testosterone is a drag queen. It looks tempting at first, but if you take it back home with you, you're in for a shitty ending.

Once aromatase claws its way into your manhood, it's not something you'll be bragging about because the excess estrogen that results can lead to greater fat storage around the belly and even Gynomastia, better known as "man-boobs." (Now who's the drag queen?)

Like all the others, bioidentical testosterone also accumulates in the fatty tissues. This sends a message to the brain that naturally-produced testosterone (the real stuff that makes you the man you are) is no longer needed and masculinity goes downhill from there. Wives might soon learn that they aren't the only chick in the marriage. Not only is excess crying a possibility, but so is insulin resistance, Type II diabetes and heart disease. Okay, I'm exaggerating about the crying part.

In 2010, *The New York Times* shined a spotlight on the risks associated with bioidentical testosterone, reporting that:

> *"A federally financed study to see if testosterone gel helps frail elderly men build muscle and strength was abruptly halted late last year after participants taking it suffered a disproportionate number of heart attacks and other serious cardiac problems."*

Even today, the FDA has not approved testosterone for those who show low levels as they age. It is strictly for use in men with hypogonadism, where sex glands produce extremely low amounts of the sex hormone, or none at all, because of an underlying disorder.

While bioidentical hormones are a safer alternative to Hormone Replacement Therapy (HRT), they are not a treatment option to be used a-la-carte for people who might be showing "low" levels of any given hormone, due to their potential risks and ability to induce hormone ignorance over time.

Chapter 2: Hormone Intelligence – The Holy Grail of Fitness, Health & Youth

My personal experience and in-depth research proved that it can be easy to "lose weight" on various fad diets. Anyone who can muster the short term willpower can become skinny through starvation and/or excessive exercise. Taking part in calorically restrictive hCG, vegan or vegetarian diets can also produce weight loss. Heck, even one Twinkie per day would drop the pounds.

But the results of these programs are rarely lasting. The initial weight loss is almost always short term and the participants in these programs usually end up fatter than they were before, with less muscle.

In fact, the underlying message of The Eight Weight Loss Lies is that "weight loss" by itself is not a measure of success.

Just consider the difference between a highly trained athlete and a couch potato, who are the same height and weight. Despite registering the same number on the scale, the appearance of these two people will be completely different. The athlete will look lean and ripped, while the couch potato will be soft and flabby.

That's why your goal should be to improve your **body composition** by eliminating fat, while building lean muscle – looking better naked. And you should do this in a way that promotes health and longevity.

The only proven and sustainable way to do this over the long term is by mastering your own hormone output, balance and sensitivity. The medical literature proves it and my own results provide the perfect example.

But it wasn't until a simple blood test showed that I had high levels of insulin and the testosterone levels of a 13-year old girl that I began to make the connection between my own "hormonal ignorance" and my growing obesity.

I didn't suffer from any specific illness, but at 30% body fat, statistics showed that I was headed toward today's top killers. These observations altered my entire view of healing, because they forced me to look for cures internally. My own research in the lab taught me that the body can provide its own pharmacy, and outside of emergency medicine, this is the only true source of healing.

Three Biological Shortcomings to Watch Out For

As a medicinal chemist, one of my tasks was to design new drugs that could mimic the effects of natural hormones when they failed to do their job among sick patients. This taught me some valuable lessons and even caused a paradigm shift in my beliefs about medicine and health.

First and foremost, I learned that just as no two fingerprints are alike, no two people share the same hormonal output, balance or sensitivity. Every man and woman have their own unique profile!

My body's output of testosterone and the ratio of it to other hormones – as well as my sensitivity to those variables – is different than anyone else's on the planet. And so is yours.

Proper hormone function isn't about the amount of hormones you have in your bloodstream, but rather how balanced they are and how sensitive you are to them!

This is in direct contrast to the myopic thinking which asserts that we need increased amounts of hormones as we age due to naturally declining levels. Far more important, is our sensitivity to hormones and their proper balance in relation to each other, as our so-called "optimal levels" begin to fall. This is why blood tests for hormone levels do not indicate hormone activity, and also the reason why raising one specific hormone with bioidenticals or otherwise fails to correct anything.

This was the most valuable lesson I learned in the laboratories of Big Pharma, because it taught me that while today's pandemic killers may exhibit different symptoms, they share the same three biological shortcomings:

1. Poor Hormone Output

2. Poor Hormone Balance

3. Poor Hormone Sensitivity

Here are a few quick examples, which show this in action.

- **Cancer patients** suffer from an imbalance of testosterone and estrogen. When the genetic map, DNA, of a single cell has been compromised by a foreign invader or toxin, it's pre-programmed to destroy itself. But due to the imbalance of sex hormones, this protective mechanism fails, causing growth and division among damaged cells. Eventually this uncontrolled cell growth compromises organ function and ultimately leads to early death as cancer runs its course internally.

- In those with **Type II diabetes**, the blood swells with excess insulin and patients become insensitive to the overload, while becoming deficient in the hormone glucagon. At the same time, estrogen and testosterone are wildly skewed.

- When **heart disease** invades our cardiovascular system, visceral fat (the fat that accumulates around your organs) begins to work against us. Inciting a hormonal storm of sorts, it throws gasoline on the inflammatory fire by producing heart attack and stroke inducing compounds known as interleukin (IL)-6, tumor necrosis factor-α (TNF-α), macrophage chemoattractant protein-1 (MCP-1), and resistin. While these words are difficult to spell, their actions in the body have been easily defined by scientists. The slew of hormones can cause inflammation and blockages within the spaghetti sized arteries of the heart, lowering blood flow and oxygen distribution.

Your Internal Pharmacy Corrects Hormonal Ignorance

To simplify the complex hormonal conundrums that I found to exist in all illnesses, I began to refer to these internal attacks as "hormonal ignorance." And despite the fact that Big Pharma was writing my paychecks at the time, my research clearly showed that hormonal ignorance can only be healed by our own body and the internal pharmacy within, rather than medications and man-made hormonal mimics!

For example:

- Cancer risk diminishes as testosterone production corrects estrogen dominance

- Type II diabetes is snuffed out when the body produces a fat burning hormone known as glucagon, and

- The threat of heart disease wanes as the body produces hormones that control blood pressure and even compensate for reduced blood flow among inflamed arteries.

The fact that our internal hormonal pharmacy can heal is in direct opposition to the commonly held views about health and healing. Most people are convinced that they need to obtain medicine from their doctor in order to heal. The truth is that the body can make its own, unique medicines specific to the individual!

This gave me hope toward my own goals of obtaining my best body. But it still didn't tell me how to actually tap into this God-given pharmacy. Not until I understood the actions of insulin in response to my own eating habits was I able to learn how to harness hormone intelligence… and hormone intelligence therapy was born.

Getting My Testosterone Back

You've heard me talk about insulin as the chief fat storing hormone, but it does a lot more than inflate your belly. During normal function, it helps increase muscle mass and acts as a taxi to shuttle nutrients and sugar out of the blood and into the muscles.

But, as I showed in great detail in my book, *Over-The-Counter Natural Cures*, insulin can wreak havoc metabolically when blood levels get too high from excess sugar and artificial flavor intake. And looking at my own eating habits, I was consuming sugar every time I put something in my mouth.

Whether I was drinking a "sports drink", eating a "health food" bar, snacking on yogurt, enjoying a bagel, beef jerky or even Campbell's soup, I was shocked to learn that I was choking down some type of detrimental sugar – sucrose, fructose, high-fructose corn syrup, dextrose, lactose, maltose and/or monosodium glutamate (MSG)!

I call these health impostors, Grocery Store Fat Traps, and as a result of my steady diet of these foods and drinks, my annual sugar consumption was about 130 pounds per year. The average American gulps down 160 pounds per year, compared to our healthier ancestors who consumed only about 10 pounds!

Little did I know I was headed toward more treacherous health problems than just obesity. I was accelerating to my own death because I was becoming "insulin resistant."

Grocery Store Fat Traps Steal My Abs and Willpower

"Insulin resistance" is a description for what happens when muscle cells resist the glucose (sugar) and nutrient delivery actions of insulin, causing blood sugar to soar. The normal range for fasting blood sugar is 85–95 ng/dl. But when insulin resistance sets in, levels spike to 110–125. That's the start of hormonal ignorance.

Like an alcoholic who has to consume more drinks to get the same intoxicating results, the pancreas responds to higher blood sugar by unleashing greater amounts of insulin to force feed the muscles. But the cells continue to resist the sugar push. Chemically, the tidal wave of insulin causes receptors to get "gummed-up." The muscle cells fail to vacuum sugar from the blood in response to the actions of insulin – a process known as **phosphorylation is no longer effective at protecting the body from high sugar levels**.

Without sugar and nutrients entering muscle cells, hormonal dynamics that control metabolism and health go AWOL. The hormones **ghrelin, leptin and cholecystokinin** fail to work in an orchestra-like unison to regulate hunger, appetite, food intake, and the feeling of being full.

Ultimately, our hormone receptors become incapable of recognizing their hormone counterparts, and metabolism comes to a screeching halt as blood sugar and insulin levels rise. Our willpower becomes wiped out and the brain screams eat, eat eat... we start eating way too fucking much while the body does nothing but store, store store.

Over time, appetite and food intake can diminish, but hormonal ignorance will continue to prevent weight loss, as calories consumed continue to be packed away as visceral fat. As you may remember, this is the abdominal fat which accumulates around your organs. This is the most dangerous type of fat, because it "oozes" inflammatory chemicals, which fuel the flames of heart disease.

As hormonal ignorance dominates, human growth hormone (hGH) fails to preserve the skin and muscle tone, and a host of other hormonal systems fizzle out, making us candidates for high blood pressure, Type II diabetes, cancer, stroke and heart attack. The output and balance of testosterone and your sensitivity to it also dissipates.

This hormonal nightmare is a global phenomenon that affects hundreds of millions worldwide and can eliminate decades from our lifespan. We are now living in the first generation of man where life expectancy is moving backwards because of insulin resistance.

My first question was, "Am I doomed to hormonal ignorance?"

I immediately got off all Grocery Store Fat Traps. I ransacked my house and trashed anything with ingredients that ended in -ose (fructose, sucrose, maltose, and such). I also started reading nutrition labels more carefully and if the ingredient list carried more than four additives, I didn't eat it.

My shelves were restocked with nutrient-rich calories – as you'll soon learn about – and I swore off my Mountain Dew vice forever. Later, I replaced it with the healthy alternative Mountain Zevia (*www.zevia.com*) and the energizing tea known as yerba mate (*www.guayaki.com*). Using my Death By Sugar Calculator (*www.sugarmeasurements.com*), I reduced my sugar intake from 130 pounds per year to 5 pounds!

Miraculous things happened...

I descended from 30% body fat to a lean 12% body fat in 90 days, living by the rule, "if it tastes sweet, spit it out." I also gained twelve pounds of muscle and my productivity, physical and mental endurance was at an all-time high. Blood tests showed my insulin and glucose levels had nosedived, while testosterone soared. And even better, the physical changes showed that my hormones were being balanced and my body was becoming more sensitive to them!

All this, and I didn't have to use any type of testosterone creams, gels, injections or pills! Thank you, God!

I felt like my discovery was the Holy-Grail for effortless fat loss and vibrant health. I began to refer to my own, physical evolution as **Hormone Intelligence Therapy (HIT)** and was officially the first HIT Man! I awoke from my metabolic nightmare and freed myself from hormonal ignorance to finally live energized and fit thanks to my own internal pharmacy working day and night to grant me better health and a physique to match.

Controlling Your Own Hormone Intelligence

With a sugar addiction behind me, it proved that my body was able to tap into its own internal pharmacy to reverse damage. I proved that hormone intelligence can be easily achieved with nothing more than a change of habits.

But what else could help me alter my hormones for the better?

I began to look for other ways to slow the aging process, boost muscle growth and improve my health through hormone intelligence. After all, longevity and hormones go hand in hand, as proven by the fact that across virtually all species, those that secrete the most insulin over a lifetime have the shortest lifespan. In fact, "perceived age" studies have even shown that people with high blood sugar levels look years older than those with low levels.

Since eating is such an integral part of our lives, I decided to investigate the almighty calorie – that elusive and sorely misunderstood staple of our diets — which is often blamed for putting us into fatter pants. "How could something so beneficial be so harmful?" I pondered. And no doubt, there are as many viewpoints on calorie-intake as there are fad diets.

Though we are so advanced in so many areas, the irony is that most people have not learned how to eat right. The only way to do so is to look closely at the effects that various types of calories and their quantities have on our biochemistry, hormones and most importantly, our DNA.

The Truth about the Calorie and how it optimizes Hormone function

Sixty-five years of studying the eating habits of mammals shows that a caloric deficit is the only proven way to slow down the aging process and increase longevity, while positively affecting hormone activity and subsequently physique. In other words, we have to stop eating so fucking much.

I'll get to the improvements in hormone intelligence and physique in a moment. And don't worry, you won't have to starve yourself!

But first, let's discuss the results related to life-extension, many of which are extraordinary. In fact, animal experiments have shown that as little as a 30% reduction in caloric intake from the baseline of normal caloric needs (while ensuring adequate micronutrient intake) can extend longevity by 40% to 50%!

The Biomedical Journal, *Natural Medicine* writes:

> *"Caloric restriction is the only intervention consistently shown to extend both median and maximal life span in mammals."*

These studies show that caloric restriction can produce the following results:

- Suppression of oxidative damage and better maintenance of antioxidant defense systems

- Less inflammation and stronger anti-inflammatory processes

- Genes involved in detoxification, antioxidant defense and enzyme repair systems were selectively up-regulated

Any one of these results would improve your health and longevity. All of them together equates to a veritable Fountain of Youth. But the greatest benefits to your health and longevity lie in our DNA, the genetic map found within the biochemical core of every cell.

Preserving Your Genetic Code

Every time your cells divide, a small portion of your DNA is lost. This is the shoe-string section at the end of the chromosome, called the telomere. As you age, the telomere gets shorter and shorter. Finally, it disappears and the cell stops dividing and dies.

Physical aging occurs as more and more cells reach the end of their telomeres and die. As the process accelerates, your muscles get weaker, wrinkles appear and eyesight fades. Eventually the organs begin to fail and death occurs. That's the nature of life.

You cannot avoid your telomeres becoming shorter as time goes by. But the good news is that your habits and lifestyle can dramatically influence the speed at which it occurs. And one of the best ways to slow the process down dramatically is to restrict the number of calories you consume.

Think of it just like the wear and tear you might put on a car. The true "age" of your car has very little to do with the number of years that go by since it was manufactured. After all, a car can sit in the garage for many years and still run like new and have its entire useful life ahead of it. On the other hand, a two-year-old car which has been driven every day and has 150,000 miles on the odometer might be near the end of its useful life.

In other words, it has little to do with the chronological age of the car... and everything to do with the number of miles and the amount of fuel the car has burned during that time. The same is true for your body. The more calories and times you eat, the faster you age. That's because they are fuel, and the more fuel you burn or energy that you consume, the greater the wear and tear on your biochemistry. That is why dozens of peer reviewed studies have shown that calorie restriction is the only tried and true, proven way to increase active longevity – it's a form of preservation.

If you're like me, you probably have mixed emotions about this research. After all, I'm sure you love food and don't care for the notion of going through the rest of your life with hunger pangs. In fact, when I first discovered this research my thoughts went back to the miserable starvation diets I endured during my collegiate wrestling days. But, it's not like that. You don't have to go through life eating like a bird and constantly racked with hunger to enjoy an extra 10 or 20 years of healthy longevity. The key is to understand nutrient and caloric density.

Nutrient Density vs. Caloric Density

Caloric restriction doesn't mean that you have to go hungry. By choosing foods that are nutrient dense versus calorie dense, you'll never have to consider the amount of calories you're consuming. Your own body will ensure that you naturally eat within a calorie range that mimics caloric restriction.

More on that in a moment... but first, what are "nutrient dense" foods?

The concept is very simple. Nutrient dense foods are those that have a high nutritional value, relative to their number of calories. For example, a grass-fed steak, an apple, or a stalk of broccoli, all have a very high level of nutrition, compared to a modest number of calories. Whole eggs, meat, fish, fruits and vegetables, nuts, berries, seeds, butter and coconut oil are all nutrient dense foods.

By contrast, a bag of potato chips or a can of soda have very few nutrients, compared to a high number of calories. Pasta, cakes, cookies, crackers, bread, cereal, food bars and most desserts are also nutrient-depleted, calorie-dense foods.

Is Sugar Threatening Your Hormones and Longevity?

To measure the impact your sugar consumption is having on your health, use the People's Chemist Death By Sugar Calculator:

www.sugarmeasurements.com

Step 1

All you have to do is measure your current daily intake in grams, by reading your labels and measuring portions for a 24 hour period.

Step 2

Insert that number into the calculator and it will calculate how many pounds of sugar you consume annually.

The bar graph will show your relative risk of disease and premature aging.

When you eat foods that are high in calories but low in nutrients, your body will continue to produce cravings for more food, despite the fact that you may have already eaten three times the number of calories you really need. On the other hand, nutrient dense foods will provide all the nutrition your body needs to ensure that your hormones keep you "feeling satisfied," even if the number of calories is considerably low. **This is the key to successfully stop eating so fucking much.**

The equation is simple:

- **Low Nutrient Density** = Food cravings, even after far too many calories

- **High Nutrient Density** = Appetite subsides, even with a significant calorie deficit

But to complete your understanding, it's critical that you know what "hunger" really means and how to control it. After all, it is virtually impossible to lose weight when your hunger is out of control. And if you are ever going to stop your cravings, you have to know where they come from.

Understanding and Controlling the Four Different Types of Hunger

There are four types of hunger. Three of them are liars. And telling obese people to "eat less" is a huge disservice of you don't teach them about the tricksters.

Most people think that hunger has everything to do with your stomach. When there is food in your belly, you feel full. When your stomach is empty, you feel hungry. This is what I call, **physical hunger**.

Physical hunger is the feeling you get several hours after a meal, after a long day of work, or after an intense exercise session. Your stomach growls and you might feel tired, irritable and have difficulty thinking. This is caused by your body's true physical need for nutrients and energy.

But your feelings of hunger are affected by many factors beyond whether your stomach is full or empty. In fact, we often feel "hungry" again, soon after a big meal. Or we experience sudden, strong cravings, especially for sweets and carbs. This is what I call **hormonal hunger**, and it has little to do with how much you've eaten and everything to do with hormonal ignorance. The cravings caused by hormonal hunger can overcome even the staunchest willpower, and can lead to intense mood swings, fatigue, and a near constant desire to eat.

Most people who consume the Standard American Diet (SAD) also experience **nutritional hunger**. This is actually another form of hormonal hunger, caused by a lack of vital nutrients. When your diet consists largely of grain-based carbohydrates and other processed, refined foods, your body is missing out on hundreds of critical vitamins, minerals, phytonutrients and enzymes. As a means of survival, it will continue to send hormonal signals to your brain to

"EAT, EAT, EAT," even when you have consumed far more calories than you need for basic energy requirements.

And finally, there is **learned hunger**. Since eating elicits a flood of feel-good molecules, the brain will "learn" when and how the food was obtained as a survival method to obtain more in the future. In its most benign form, learned hunger arises at meal time. And since 1pm – lunchtime – comes around only once per day, its fine.

But, in its most malignant form, learned hunger can force someone into overeating based simply on bad eating habits. For instance. if someone eats multiple times per day (bodybuilders and athletes) or while watching television, learned hunger can set in and force them to become hungry each and every time the situation presents itself. Athletes who eat every two hours, are simply training their body to become hungry despite no need for nutrients. Same for children – or anyone else – who eat in front of the television. Subconsciously, associations will be made based on learned hunger and forced overeating.

You see, the hunger that most people feel has nothing to do with a real need for food, most of the time your hormones or brain are lying to you. It is either caused by the body's demand for nutrients, raging hormones of hunger or learned hunger.

Understanding how the three types of hunger can fool us shows why it's not fair or prudent to tell overweight people to simply eat less – it's virtually impossible without teaching them about "the right calories" and how these foods help to control your anti-hunger hormones and promote a long-lasting feeling of fullness. These powerful urges can be eliminated by choosing nutrient-dense foods that promote hormone intelligence, at the right times of the day.

I'm talking about eggs, butter, whey... grass-fed beef, pastured pork and poultry... wild fish... a wide variety of vegetables and fruit... nuts, seeds and berries... and select nutritional supplements.

Not only are these foods slowly digested, but they are also rich in healthy fats and protein, which will keep you full much longer than processed carbohydrates. These are the foods that will truly nourish your body and enhance your metabolism as you will learn in the upcoming habits.

But it's vital that you know that as long as you learn to choose the "right calories," your body will produce and become more sensitive to anti-hunger hormones. These chemical messengers trick your brain into thinking the stomach is full.

In contrast, if you choose the wrong calories, you can be haunted by the same hunger and cravings that haunted me as a college wrestler trying to make weight.

The bottom line is: Don't count calories – make your calories count!

With caloric restriction pointing the way to more youthful DNA (longer telomeres) and a longer life, I wondered about athletic performance. Did my hormonal ignorance change the way my body responded to exercise? Of course it did, so I set out to change it. And a military training tactic called "blood loading" showed me how.

Making of the Elite Soldier and Athlete

In their pursuit of soldiers with ultra-endurance and strength, the US military learned how to spike strength and endurance hormones in record time by tapping into our body's own "internal pharmacy."

Through trial and error they found that cadets who trained at high altitude performed far better when they got back to sea level. The effect was magnified using a diet enhanced with naturally occurring amino acids, iron, vitamin B12, folate and minerals such as zinc, copper, vitamin A, B-complex, thermogenic aids (compounds that activate fat metabolism) and vitamin C.

Upon blood analysis, it was discovered that the performance enhancing effect was the result of a special family of cells that utilized these nutrients to manufacture hormones like hGH, testosterone, glucagon and an oxygen carrying hormone known as hemoglobin. The high elevation forced the cadet's bodies to adapt by improving their hormone intelligence.

The blood of the training soldiers was so rich in these adaptive hormones that medical teams were able to extract it, store it and then re-inject it later to maximize performance on the battlefield! As higher levels of testosterone, growth hormone, glucagon and hemoglobin surged through their blood, soldiers instantly attained keen focus as well as greater strength and endurance.

Their lean body mass was also drastically increased, as body fat plummeted and functional muscle was added. Hearts were strengthened and the cardio-vascular system worked more efficiently (as measured by a lower resting heart rate). Metabolism was super-charged with anabolic hormones that decreased appetite and forced the body to make better use of nutrients.

These outcomes led to the making of elite soldiers and ultimately became a top-secret technique known as "blood loading." When done under the keen supervision of doctors, it showed to be safer and more effective than man-made drugs used in Hormone Replacement Therapy (HRT) and even so-called Bioidentical Hormone Replacement Therapy (BHRT).

While negative side effects of blood loading are possible, the technique highlights the fact that the real source of man's performance-enhancement comes from our own internal pharmacy!

The studies on caloric deficiencies and the making of elite soldiers – along with my own results as a HIT Man – prove that it is our habits, not our inheritance that shape the function and actions of our DNA and subsequently our hormone intelligence.

This becomes even clearer as you watch certain family members either lose their health or gain it, relative to others as they change their habits or adhere to destructive family traditions. The same is true across cultures.

The same intelligence that puts our internal pharmacy into motion to automatically control breathing, heart rate, body temperature and the removal of waste products, as well as to sharpen the endurance of soldiers who took part in "blood loading" experiments can also help you become a HIT Man or Woman.

Chapter 3: Six Habits to Becoming a HIT Man or Woman

By adhering to Hormone Intelligence Therapy, people of all body types, race, gender and age can live relatively thin and slim. That's because all living cells carry the DNA blueprint that dictates hormone intelligence based on habits, which you are to never forget, is:

1. Optimal Hormone Output

2. Optimal Hormone Balance

3. Optimal Hormone Sensitivity

As others learned of my findings and applied them, they too achieved their optimal weight and physique, while attaining vibrant health, energy and mental clarity as HIT Men and Women. And it is no surprise when you learn how capable our internal pharmacy really is...Take a few minutes to review this partial list of hormones that begin working in your favor as a HIT Man or Woman (Table 2).

Table 2: Your Internal Pharmacy

Hormone	Action	Increased Activity	Decreased Activity
Human Growth Hormone	Builds muscle, burns fat, responsible for maintaining youth, strength and health	Explosive exercise movements. Workouts that focus on the largest muscle groups. Deep, restful sleep also raises levels.	Lack of sleep, or going to bed too late, sugar and artificial flavor intake, long duration endurance exercise, chronic stress
Testosterone	Along with hGH builds muscle mass and strength. Helps prevent increases in body fat. Plays a role in bone strength. Normal levels maintain mood and confidence.	Heavy weight lifting, earlier bedtimes and normal sleep, Avoid environmental estrogens Keep body fat down	Obesity, insulin resistance, diabetes, belly fat, inactivity
Estrogen	Maintains bone density, female reproductive system, supports blood vessel function. Estrogen dominance can increase subcutaneous body fat ("thunder thighs")	High Body Fat Perimenopausal estrogen surges Pregnancy Liver dysfunction Excess meals In men – high aromatase levels	Menopause, extreme dieting, anorexia nervosa, excessive endurance exercise. High intake of phytoestrogens (esp soy), environmental estrogens (such as plastic, pesticides) will interfere with natural estrogen function
Leptin	Produced by adipocytes, in response to increase in fat storage, decreases hunger/appetite and stimulates increase in physical activity. Regulates weight on day-to-day basis in normal weight individuals.	Short term weight gain in response to transient overeating in "normal weight" individuals increases leptin along with proper signaling Long term weight gain and obesity cause very high leptin levels, interferes with signaling, and therefore leptin resistance	Obesity results in high production but reduced sensitivity. Extreme weight loss can depress leptin production encouraging rebound weight gain.

Hormone	Action	Increased Activity	Decreased Activity
Ghrelin	Released in stomach during fasting state. Increases hunger. Also stimulates Growth Hormone release	Empty Stomach Diet-induced weight loss Low leptin levels Sleep deprivation – may initially decrease ghrelin, then rebound increase occurs later in day	Full stomach Obesity (sometimes) Hyperinsulinemia High leptin levels Exercise (short term decreases in ghrelin and appetite)
Catecholamines	*Epinephrine (adrenaline)* – stimulates glycogen breakdown into blood glucose (energy for flight or fight), increased heart rate, increases BMR *Dopamine* – Feel good neurotransmitter, motivating, precursor to norepinephrine which is precursor to epinephrine	*Epinephrine* Stress, Stimulants such as caffeine and certain herbs *Dopamine* – exercise, may be at least partially responsible for "runners high", nicotine (not recommended!)	*Epinephrine*: Fatigue, overstimulation leading to "adrenal burnout", rebound decrease in production *Dopamine* – low protein intake (phenylalanine is precursor), diseases such as Parkinson's
Thyroid Hormones	Regulates metabolic rate via active form triiodothyronine T3, bone mineralization via calcitonin	Proper intake of iodide (too much or too little causes goiter), adequate intake of micronutrients that convert T4 to T3	Iodide deficiency, low calorie diets, goitrogens in soy, raw cruciferous vegetables, autoimmune disease, lack of nutrients that enable conversion of T4 to T3

Hormone	Action	Increased Activity	Decreased Activity
Serotonin	Induces feelings of well being and contentment Low serotonin levels increase cravings for carbohydrate	Carbohydrate intake helps the amino acid tryptophan convert to serotonin, Neuropeptide Y elevated in the morning when serotonin levels are low – eating breakfast (carbs) restores serotonin	Low levels of neuropeptide Y, low levels of tryptophan found in animal protein, Stress may deplete serotonin
Cortisol	Increases release of glucose into blood, partly via catabolizing muscle mass for gluconeogenesis, glucose then stored as fat, reduced bone mineral density	Lack of sleep can prevent diurnal decrease (however high cortisol might be cause of insomnia), chronic psychological and/or physical stress (such as excessive cardio)	Deep breathing and meditation, vitamin C from citrus fruits, low glycemic load diet, Possibly magnesium
Adiponectin	Produced by adipocytes, Increases insulin sensitivity, allows muscle cells to use glucose for energy	Exercise, especially resistance Increase in omega-3 fatty acids (possibly)	Obesity Low intake of omega-3 (possibly)
PYY	Appetite suppressant released after meals in intestines	Protein intake	Low protein intake, obese people may also produce less
Glucagon	Glycogen breakdown to restore optimal blood glucose levels,liberates fat from adipocytes, however also muscle protein breakdown for gluconeogenesis	Skipping meals, low carb diets,exercise Glucagon beneficial for weight loss to a degree, continued secretion can cause protein breakdown for energy	High glycemic load diets,because glucagon cannot be elevated if insulin levels are high Lack of exercise
Insulin	Uptake of blood glucose by cells for energy production, synthesis of liver and muscle glycogen, muscle protein synthesis, fat storage.	Low-fat, high carbohydrate diet, particularly refined carbs	Eliminate refined carbs, balanced low glycemic diets, dietary fats and oils increase CCK and slow glucose absorption, exercise

Hormone	Action	Increased Activity	Decreased Activity
Cholecystokinin	The "satiety" hormone, slows down the rate at which food leaves the stomach, reduces glycemic response, normalizes appetite	Presence of fat, and to a lesser degree protein, in stomach.	Low-fat, high-carbohydrate diets.
Amylin	Secreted at the same time as insulin by same pancreatic cells, it reduces rate of gastric emptying and glucose absorption, reducing appetite	Eating	Obesity can result in high production leading to Amylin resistance.
IGF-1	Synergistic with Growth Hormone, mediates repair of muscle and other tissue, maintains youth, helps burn fat	Casein and whey (dairy proteins) have been shown to increase levels	Low protein intake, starvation, other catabolic conditions. Exercise might increase sensitivity.
PGC1 – Alpha	Increases mitochondria, increases synthesis of slow twitch muscle fibers, increases insulin sensitivity	Endurance exercise and interval training	Excess drug and alcohol intake, liver injury
EPO	Oxygen uptake and distribution, increases strength and endurance, increases vascularization	High altitude training, testosterone, lack of sugar	Estrogen dominance, sugar intake, low altitude training, fatigue, low testosterone
DHT	Male sex hormone, responsible for strength and muscle mass	Healthy fat intake	Sugar intake, atrophy, lack of exercise

I produced the table above to give you an idea of the many hormones that help to regulate your appetite, fat storage, metabolism, muscle-building, strength, endurance, libido… and the dietary and lifestyle habits that increase or decrease these hormones and your body's sensitivity to them.

But I don't want you to get caught up in the complexity of all of that. The great news is that you don't have to worry about any of it. Your body will naturally move toward a state of hormone intelligence, where all of these hormones (and many more) are secreted in just the right amounts… they are perfectly balanced in relation to one another… and your body is highly sensitive to each one of them.

The key is to follow the six HIT habits, below…

HIT Habit #1 – If it Tastes Sweet Spit it Out

If it tastes sweet, you have to spit it out. This includes fruit, too, among anyone who is overweight due to hormonal ignorance. If you don't stop habitually eating sweets, energy bars, cereal, ice cream and drinking sodas, sports drinks and sugary fruit juices, your body will endlessly crave these foods. It's not natural. It's not safe. And all amounts of sugar are detrimental to those who are hormonally ignorant. Some would argue that fruit is acceptable, but the sweetness that comes from the naturally occurring fructose molecule acts just like sugar among the "insulin resistant," and therefore increases fat storage, as proven with simple blood tests.

Children are not immune to sugar's metabolic turmoil either. *The medical journal Lancet* reported that children who consume even a single sugary soda per day are 60% more likely to become obese.

Quitting sugar can be difficult, because not only does it taste good, it can also be physically and emotionally addictive. The addiction is set into motion by an increase in the "feel-good" molecules known as endorphins and a subsequent lack of their precursor serotonin. Similar to a drug addiction, serotonin levels are depleted once the sugar high dissipates. Without serotonin, you feel "down and out" because you are unable to produce endorphins.

To remedy this, a sugar addict reaches for more sugar, like a cocaine addict reaches for cocaine. In fact, scientists who have studied the addictive properties of the white powders on mice, found that sugar is even more addictive than the illicit drugs!

This explains the phenomenon of "emotional eating." Without sugar, regular users are irritable, hungry and lack focus. Their "quick fix" is something sweet or a carbohydrate-rich food like bagels, chips, cereal or pretzels.

Women are more susceptible to sugar addiction than men, probably due to higher estrogen levels, which can make them more sensitive to highs and lows of blood sugar and endorphins. Plus, you can see it in action because more women than men reach for chocolate during times of stress or sadness, although it can happen to men too.

Your goal should be to keep your sugar intake below 15 pounds per year. Although less than 10 pounds annually is even better, based on population studies showing the positive relationship between low sugar intake and a healthy lifespan. Based on your current grams per day average, cut your sugar use by half the first week and then to a quarter for two weeks. After that, be done with it for good.

For example, if you currently consume an average of 120 grams of sugar per day, that's about 100 pounds per year (about 90 pounds too much)! Cut it to 60 grams per day for the first week and then 30 grams for the second and third. This would reduce your annual sugar consumption from 100 pounds to a mere 8 pounds!

This one change will be more effective at helping you feel great and keeping you alive longer than any medicine in the world!

You will be surprised how quickly your cravings subside. It won't happen overnight, but your body's innate hormone intelligence will soon take over. Within just a week or two, your appetite will be easier to control, your mood and energy levels will be more stable, and your cravings for sweets will dissipate.

Be sure to get plenty of sunlight during this period (a good idea at all times) and you may wish to supplement with the essential amino acid L-tryptophan in the evening. I have designed a product called SerotoninFX (www.thepeopleschemist. com/serotonin-fx), which contains this important compound.

Doing this will increase your body's ability to produce serotonin and can help alleviate the cravings without causing you to reach for a quick fix in the form of a soda, candy bar, dessert or other carbohydrate-rich snacks.

However, as bad as sugar can be, artificial sweeteners such as sucralose (Splenda), aspartame (Equal), acesulfame-K, saccharin and neotame are even worse. In addition to numerous health consequences, these chemical ingredients disrupt satiety (the feeling of fullness) and can alter taste receptors on the tongue that communicate flavor and caloric intake to the brain. This can cause your body to lose its natural ability to count calories and lead you to overeat without conscious awareness.

If you simply must have an occasional sweet treat, don't worry. There are plenty of healthy, natural alternatives, including stevia (plant based) and erythritol (nontoxic sugar alcohol that doesn't raise insulin or blood sugar) that you can use to create delicious desserts and sweeten your beverages without souring your health.

Stevia extract is one of the most popular natural alternatives to sugar. It's 100% safe. The stevia plant has been used for hundreds, if not thousands of years in South America, and has been used for decades in modern commercial products in Japan and Brazil. In addition to its clean, sweet taste, animal and human studies show that stevia extract can help lower systolic and diastolic blood pressure. It has also been shown to prevent and even reverse insulin resistance by helping to clear glucose from the blood stream.

You can easily find stevia online or in your local health food store. Just make sure the brand you choose does not have maltodextrin in it, which can raise blood sugar (I prefer NuStevia No Carbs Blend from *www.nunaturals.com*).

Other products that you can use, occasionally, to get your sweet fix without harming your health are Zevia brand sodas (*www.zevia.com*) and WellnessBakeries (*www.wellnessbakeries.com*) for delicious desserts.

Desserts That Won't Kill You

Finally, if you enjoy baking your own healthy desserts from scratch and don't want to harm your health indulging in them, I highly recommend the recipe book and educational program found at www.safetaste.com, which provides over 50 delicious and healthy dessert recipes (plus gluten free, low-carb breads, crusts and crepes) using exclusively safe, natural ingredients.

HIT Habit #2 – Make Purified Water Your Drink of Choice

A proven and very simple fat loss technique is water consumption. Not only will this help to curb your appetite, but scientists from Humboldt University have also confirmed that drinking water increases thermogenesis.

Utilizing a technique known as whole-room indirect calorimetry (a very accurate way to measure human energy expenditure) the researchers were able to measure the effect of drinking water on fat metabolism. What they discovered is that when the subjects of the study drank 16 ounces of water in one sitting, thermogenesis was increased by a whopping 30%!

To harness this simple fat burning technique drink 8–16 ounces of spring water, or second best, purified water (via reverse osmosis or the simple ZeroWater filter/pitcher combo available at *www.amazon.com*) when you wake up and shortly before every meal. Pant sizes will decrease.

Best water

- Reverse Osmosis

- ZeroWater Filter/Pitcher from *Amazon.com*

Don't drink your calories! Calorie rich beverages like beer, sodas, fruit juices and sports drinks do nothing to increase your fullness and can easily add a serious number of calories and sugar to your daily total. If you like the occasional energy drink, choose yerba mate tea from *www.guayaki.com*.

HIT Habit #3 – Restrict Your Calories for Hormone Intelligence, Not Starvation

Calculating your caloric need for HIT isn't an exact science. Since everyone's hormones are different, each person's reaction to them will be different. Your goal as a HIT Man or Woman is to:

- Learn how to choose the right calories

- Calculate your estimated daily caloric need based on your ideal weight

- Consume your calories as 50% healthy fat, 25% protein, 25% carbohydrates

- Only eat three times per day, no snacking

- Never drink your calories from soda, flavored water, juices or sports drinks

These rules will help you achieve a caloric deficit, without becoming hungry, aggravated or "psycho-glycemic." At first, eating only three meals per day, spaced out by five hours, might be tough because your body may be "hormonally ignorant" and not prepared to control cravings and naturally curb your hunger. However, as you gain control of your hormones, it will become progressively easier to avoid snacking.

In the next chapter, I will discuss the first step in greater detail: How to choose the right calories, in other words, which foods to enjoy and which to avoid, in order to achieve hormone intelligence and ultimately transform your body and your health without going hungry.

But for now, let me show you how to calculate the estimated number of calories you need to consume each day to preserve lean body mass, shed fat and reach your ideal weight. While choosing the right foods to consume is ultimately the most important thing, you still have to ensure that you achieve a caloric deficit to experience the most rapid and effective fat loss.

To estimate your total caloric need, you need to determine your ideal weight, then your Basal Metabolic Rate (BMR), and finally add your "activity level." It's a simple three-step process.

Step 1. Calculate your ideal weight

The best way to figure your ideal weight is by identifying the amount of fat you are lugging around, then "cut the fat in half." You can't subtract all of it because your body needs some fat to survive.

After cutting the fat in half, subtract that number from your current weight.

Example

Example for a 37 year old male, 69 inches tall, whose current weight is 205 pounds and body fat percentage is 30%:

Current body fat: 30%

Amount of fat on body = 205 x (.30) = 61.5 lbs

Cutting the fat in half (rounded): ~30 lbs

Ideal weight is 205-30 = 175 lbs

Your Ideal Weight Calculations

Body Fat %:

Amount of Fat on Body:

Cutting the Fat In Half:

Your Ideal Weight = (Current weight) − (Fat Cut In Half) =

Note: As a means of estimating ideal weight, this usually leaves 12% to 20% body fat for men, and 15% to 25% for women. The obvious flaw is that your "ideal weight" may or may not grant you with your "best body." That's because it doesn't predict how much fat will be lost or muscle gained as you reach your target. Don't worry about it...You're not putting on the bikini just yet.

The ideal weight might not be where you end up once you hit your preferred body fat percentage because you will also be putting on lean, sexy muscle. This ideal weight calculation is simply used to estimate your caloric needs. Later, I'll show you how to obtain your "best body" once you descend toward your ideal weight using "lean body mass."

Figure 1. How to calculate your ideal weight

Step 2. Use Ideal Weight to Calculate "BMR Calorie Requirement"

Now that you have your ideal weight, you will calculate how many calories your body needs for Basic Metabolic Rate (BMR). This is simply the number of calories to sustain basic physiological functions like breathing, circulation and brain activity. The formulas for men and women are below:

Men

BMR = 66 + (6.23 x ideal weight in pounds) + (12.7 x height in inches) – (6.8 x age in years)

Example	Your BMR Calorie Requirement
Example for a 37-year old male, 69 inches tall, whose ideal weight is 175 pounds:	
$66 + (6.23 \times 175) + (12.7 \times 69) - (6.8 \times 37)$	
$66 + 1090.25 + 876.3 - 251.6 = \sim1780$	
BMR Calorie Requirement = 1780 calories per day to sustain BMR	**BMR Calorie Requirement =**

Women

BMR = 655 + (4.36 x ideal weight in pounds) + (4.7 x height in inches) – (4.7 x age in years)

Example	Your BMR Calorie Requirement
Example for a 35 year old woman, 64 inches tall, whose ideal weight is 125 pounds:	
$655 + (4.36 \times 125) + (4.7 \times 64) - (4.7 \times 35)$	
$655 + 545 + 300.8 - 164.5 = 1336.3$	
BMR Calorie Requirement = 1336.3 calories per day to sustain BMR	**BMR Calorie Requirement =**

Figure 2. How to calculate BMR calorie requirement

Step 3. Add Your Activity Level to Obtain "Daily Estimated Caloric Need"

Obviously, you're going to do more than just lie in bed all day. So you have to add an "activity factor" that comes from a percentage of the total BMR. Of course, the activity factor is quite subjective. For an athlete in training, it might be 30% to 40% of BMR.

As a HIT Man or Woman, I suggest using 20%. This program is not dependent on exercise, its dependent on hormones and if you follow the upcoming exercise principles, you'll only need to work out 3 to 4 times per week.

Now, add your activity level of 20%:

BMR Calorie Requirement x Activity Level = Calories to add to BMR

Activity calories + BMR = Estimated Daily Caloric Need

Example for the male above at 20% activity level:

1780 x .20 = 356

Therefore 356 + 1780 = 2136 total daily calories

To sum it up, the estimated caloric need for a 37 year old male whose ideal weight is 175 pounds, is 2136.

Your Estimated Daily Caloric Need Calculation

(BMR)(.20) = Calories to add Activity calories + BMR = Daily Caloric Need

Daily Caloric Need =

Figure 3. How to calculate your daily caloric need

The Best Way to Get Your Daily Calories Isn't by Grazing!

Once you've determined your daily estimated caloric need, you will consume them via three daily meals, spacing each one out by about 5 hours. Your meals should be comprised of 50% fat, 25% carbohydrate and 25% protein, measured from grams (see your food labels). Don't split hairs over this. You don't need decimal point accuracy.

By following this eating frequency in these proportions you will avoid hunger, activate diet-induced thermogenesis (DIT) and simultaneously ensure that your "insulin recovery" occurs as quickly as possible after each meal. If you snack or eat more than three meals (eat too fucking often), you may slowly ignite insulin resistance and squash hormone intelligence.

Elite athletes may take in four meals per day, and even consume up to 50% in non-sweet, complex carbohydrates. But for future HIT hopefuls, 50% healthy fat is highly recommended, via three meals per day only.

Once you have reached your ideal weight and lean body mass, you can raise your complex carbohydrate intake considerably. Your ratio could look something like 40% carbohydrates, 35% healthy fats, 25% protein. Elite athletes would do something like 50% carbohydrates, 30% protein, 20% healthy fats.

Don't forget, this whole calorie calculation thing is an estimate, based on a formula that is almost one hundred years old. That means your final number may be too high or too low. So simply use this as a guide to begin planning your meals.

As you become a HIT Man or Woman, the same hormone intelligence that automatically governs metabolism, pain sensation, heart rate, circulation, and breathing will also regulate your caloric intake and appetite control. If you are having difficulty with hunger between meals, the following may be preventing you from becoming satiated:

1. You didn't eat enough at meal time.

2. Your previous meal consisted of too many carbohydrate calories and not enough healthy fat.

3. You are not exercising for hormesis (see habit #5).

4. Blood sugar regulation, liver and adrenal functions are not working properly, and need time to recoup under HIT.

5. Your digestion is being shunted. Google "$1.41 Cleanse" and do it monthly.

It will take some practice to learn how to eat enough at meal time so that you are not ravenously hungry between meals. But you will learn and your hormones will adapt.

HIT Habit #4 – Utilize Thermogenic Aids

You bought the shoes in your favorite color. You're sporting the latest workout tops to lean out your features. And you even have the iPod that'll do everything for you, except sit ups. Now get a real fat-burning boost and start using a "thermogenic aid" already!

Thermogenic aids induce heat production within the body. Like wood for a fire, the fuel for this internal inferno is belly fat! By activating a unique set of metabolic switches known as beta-receptors, thermogenic aids set into motion a cascade of hormonal events that favor fat metabolism and muscle building over fat storage and muscle wasting. Body sculpting begins.

Without a thermogenic aid, many fit-hopefuls are unable to respond to exercise and healthy eating, or at least respond to a higher degree because they have become "resistant" to their own thermogenic hormones.

Just like someone can become resistant to insulin, they can also become resistant to hormones that flip on their metabolic switches. Fortunately, researchers have discovered that certain "thermogenic" compounds like citrus aurantium, guarana, yohimbe, yerba mate and green tea re-sensitize the body to its body-sculpting hormones.

In fact, learning how to selectively activate beta-receptors with thermogenic aids (termed beta-agonists) is one of the most important scientific discoveries to date because it shows how to reverse "hormonal ignorance" among those who were previously doomed, despite their best diet and exercise efforts! It gives the obese a second chance at living thin and slim.

One of the largest studies ever performed on the use of thermogenic aids was a collaborative effort by Harvard, Columbia, New York Obesity Research Center, and the Research Department of Human Nutrition in Copenhagen, Denmark. The study found that subjects using thermogenic aids – even for a short period of time – were able to reduce body weight by up to 11 pounds of fat compared to the group not taking it. With respect to negative side effects it was noted that, "There were no significant adverse effects resulting from treatment."

The study proved that thermogenic aids were able to:

- Promote the release of fat from fat stores

- Stimulate thyroid metabolism

- Boost oxygen consumption by increasing bronchodilation (the opening of bronchial tubes)

- Enhance energy capacity due to increased blood flow to the muscles, providing for an increased supply of oxygen and nutrients

- Elevate energy, mood, motivation and concentration

That's why I designed ThermoFX. Unlike other wanna-be products, it has zero synthetic caffeine or additives and works with the body to snap your fat cells out of storage mode and force them into thermogenesis mode by making your receptors more sensitive to its metabolic hormones. Using the latest techniques in natural product chemistry, I was able to utilize the most potent, whole herb blends to offer an array of thermogenic aids in only one single pill, which has never been done.

Below is a list of Mother Nature's most potent thermogenic aids, all of which were used in the design of ThermoFX AM and ThermoFX PM products:

- **Green Tea and Citrus Aurantium** – The fat burning qualities of green tea and the herbal medicine, citrus aurantium, are attributed to their ability to activate the sympathetic nervous system (SNS). These natural ingredients increase fat loss among the obese by increasing thermogenesis. The end result is the conversion of stored fat into heat. Pregnant women and those who are nursing should not use citrus aurantium. Green tea is the better option.

- **Guarana** – Among other beneficial nutrients found in the fruit, the seeds and extracts of this climbing plant, native to the Amazon, it serves as the healthiest source of natural caffeine. Caffeine helps to increase the effectiveness of thermogenic substances by blocking the actions of adenosine. This neurotransmitter not only induces sleep, it also down-regulates the sympathetic nervous system (SNS), discouraging fat loss. By temporarily blocking the activity of adenosine, guarana extract ensures that our metabolic switches stay turned on during exercise. The quantity of caffeine used does not need to be excessive. Typically, 25 to 75 mg is sufficient to ensure continued fat loss (for reference, a cup of coffee has 90 to 150 mg). Using this small amount ensures that you do not become addicted to it or suffer from side effects like headaches – it's just enough to wake up your fat cells, without leaving you wired!

- **White Willow Bark** – White willow bark eliminates another biological event that discourages fat loss – the over-production of prostaglandins. These messenger molecules are ubiquitous within your body. And when thermogenesis is increased via the conversion of fat to energy, prostaglandin messengers communicate "stop" to fat cells. This causes fat loss to be short lived. By using the prostaglandin inhibitor known as white willow bark, you can prevent this. They ensure that the conversion of fat to energy continues to occur for a significant period of time.

Night time fat loss and appetite control can be achieved without keeping you awake. This is possible by controlling blood sugar, optimizing digestion and preventing the conversion of carbohydrates to fat.

- **Apple Cider Vinegar** – Hippocrates (the 'Father of Medicine') treated his patients in 400 B.C with apple cider vinegar (ACV). He discovered that ACV is a powerful cleansing and healing elixir, as well as a naturally occurring antibiotic and antiseptic that fights germs and bacteria. ACV can also be used to prevent energy imbalance after a meal. Like vitamin C it normalizes the insulin and blood sugar response to meals. It also helps to prevent overeating. Combined, the actions of ACV work to prevent excess fat storage while you sleep.

- **Garcinia Cambogia** – This plant-based medicine contains hydroxycitric acid (HCA), which has been shown to inhibit the biosynthesis of fatty acids from carbohydrate and sugar consumption. Therefore, consumption of garcinia cambogia effectively reduces fat storage at night.

- **Cayenne** – This is among the best natural products for maximizing health and increasing thermogenesis. The synergistic effect of the active ingredients, including capsaicin, have been well documented to help convert fat to heat without stimulation. Cayenne has also been used for centuries to aid digestion, ease muscle pain, relieve headaches, reduce arthritis pain and prevent the formation of blood clots that trigger heart attacks.

- **Ginger Root** – Ginger root has long been known as nature's best anti-nausea and anti-emitive (vomiting) medicine. It has been shown to improve circulation and prevent motion sickness. The active ingredients responsible for these effects (phenylalkylketones and volatile oils) improve your body's ability to digest food and deliver nutrients for proper energy output and appetite control.

- **Bromelain** – This naturally occurring digestive enzyme is found in pineapple. When consumed, it has a very similar action to that of our own digestive enzymes produced and released by the pancreas. Supplementing with bromelain ensures that solid food is effectively broken down and properly converted into energy producing substrates.

HIT Habit #5 – Sleep Like a Drunken Bum Naturally

When your body does not get enough deep sleep, biochemical changes occur which lead to the storage of fat. The disruption of normal sleep patterns can cause insulin to rise and increase your cravings for food the following day, especially sweets.

To burn fat and maintain a lean, sexy body, it is imperative that you get plenty of sleep! One very important reason is that your production of human growth hormone – your body's internal "Fountain of Youth" – is highly dependent on deep, restful sleep. In fact, there is a major surge of growth hormone that occurs during the first 30–60 minutes after falling asleep. But this output can be aborted when your sleep is fitful and disrupted.

Consumption of carbohydrates can also disturb your night time hGH output. Carbs in your belly when you go to bed will raise your blood sugar and insulin and cause your body to abort the secretion of growth hormone. Studies show that fasting for a few hours prior to sleep can heighten sleep-related growth hormone output. At the very least, refrain from consuming carbohydrates within 90 minutes of going to bed.

Making deep sleep a high priority in your life will also help you to relieve stress and the storage of fat that can result. Stress comes in many forms. It can be physical, like an injury or illness. Or it can be mental, like problems in your career, relationships and finances. Whatever the underlying cause, feelings of stress cause the hormones cortisol and insulin to rise and fat storage to go up.

To ensure that you sleep like a drunken bum, without drinking your body weight in wine, consider the fast-acting herbal tea, California Poppy (*www.starwest-botanicals.com*). Brew ½ to 1 full cup in a French press, then enjoy. Not only will it knock you out, but it can also create a pleasant euphoric feeling, which helps keep your mind off daily stressors as you're aiming for shut-eye.

You may also consider an extremely effective product that I created, called SerotoninFX, containing a blend of valerian root and the amino acid, L-tryptophan (*http://thepeopleschemist.com/serotonin-fx*). Take one capsule per 75lbs of body weight about an hour before bedtime. Within 45 minutes you should be feeling drowsy and relaxed. It's the most potent, natural sleep aid ever!

And don't forget, stress can also come from negative people who don't support your health goals. They may invalidate you or question the changes you are making in your life. If you listen to them, they win, so don't fall for it. Just stick to your goals and let your results speak for themselves. Don't bother trying to change anyone's mind or explain **HIT** to them.

The only way for someone to learn about HIT is to study it on their own. The only thing they need to know is that you are optimizing the hormones in your body for living young, and looking great as a HIT Man or Woman.

HIT Habit #6 – Exercise to Activate Hormesis

I started running when I was 10 years old. Officially, it was my first form of exercise. Thanks to my fifth grade P.E. teacher, I was constantly competing in two-mile races after school. It hurt like hell and left me feeling nauseous and dizzy for a few minutes afterwards. But without fail, at about the 10-minute recovery mark, I always felt the warm rush of endorphins. I've been hooked ever since.

I didn't know it at the time, but the "runners high" I experienced, and the pain-soothing, euphoria inducing endorphins that caused it, was the result of a complex biological process called hormesis.

Whatever Doesn't Kill You Makes You Stronger
The word "hormesis" is derived from a Greek word, which means to stimulate or to set into motion. It is an evolutionary adaptive response, whereby a positive and beneficial result is achieved from low-dose exposure to an agent that is toxic or even lethal at higher doses.

Your body's response to sun exposure is an example of hormesis. If you were to spend too much time in the sun or get a severe sunburn, it can be very damaging and painful, and in extreme cases, life threatening. But moderate and consistent sun exposure is one of the most powerful and beneficial ways to boost your health.

Or consider trace metals, for example. There are a number of trace metals that are vital to your diet and improve your health, when consumed in "trace" amounts. And yet many of these same substances are toxic at higher levels.

The stress that is caused by physical exertion is another example. When you over-exert your body or engage in chronic endurance exercise, it can wear down your immune system, lead to extreme fatigue, and cause oxidative and inflammatory damage to your body. It also creates a hormonal state where your body chooses to store fat and tear down muscle. Not exactly the results you were hoping for from your exercise routine!

But when you exercise the right way (which you'll discover exactly how to do below with the HIT Exercise Principles), the effects are just the opposite. You will improve your immune system and promote an anti-inflammatory state. You will also create a hormonal environment in your body that leads to expanded lung volume, greater oxygen-carrying capacity of the blood, a stronger heart, more muscle and less fat.

Your goal with exercise is to harness the biological phenomenon of hormesis to produce positive adaptive changes. Anything else is just a waste of time, or worse, a waste of health.

An **adaptive response** is a change that your body makes after confronting a challenge. This is a survival mechanism that's hardwired into your genetics.

The way you do that is not by working out for a longer period of time. Rather, it is about challenging your peak capacity, even for a brief moment. When you push yourself near your maximum capacity, your body doesn't know if you're doing calisthenics in the back yard or escaping from a tiger in the jungle.

Either way, as soon as the period of physical stress has ended, your body will immediately unleash an entire pharmacy of hormones, altering your biochemistry. These messenger molecules send powerful signals to stimulate muscle development, eliminate fat, and increase the capacity of your heart and lungs. That way, you are better equipped to survive the next potential encounter in the "jungle."

What it really means, is that you won't be embarrassed to strip down at the beach anymore!

Recapping the Six Habits Of HIT

By now, you should understand exactly what "hormone intelligence" is. And you also know how to achieve it, by following the **Six HIT Habits to Becoming a HIT Man or Woman**.

Just to recap, here they are:

1. If it tastes sweet, spit it out

2. Make purified water your drink of choice

3. Restrict your calories for hormone intelligence, not starvation

4. Use thermogenic aids

5. Sleep like a drunken bum naturally

6. Exercise to activate hormesis

But there are even more vital details about what foods you should eat to boost your hormone intelligence, and which foods you should avoid at all costs. And I want to show you the right way to exercise to activate hormesis and optimize your body's hormonal output, balance and sensitivity. That's what we'll cover in the next two sections.

Chapter 4: How to Choose the Right Calories

As we discussed earlier, a calorie is simply a unit of measure – like horsepower – that defines how much energy is generated from a given food when burned. To measure this energy, a device known as a calorimeter is used.

However, unlike a calorimeter, the human body is quite complex and doesn't treat all calories the same. Not to mention, it looks way better in a bikini! While some foods can have the same caloric content, they can have vastly different effects on your hormones. Therefore, you can't measure whether a food is good or bad, simply based on "how many calories" it has.

For example, a gram of carbohydrates has about four calories, while a gram of naturally occurring fat has about nine calories. Based largely on this observation, the USDA advised the world that fat is bad and converted most of us into grain-eating "carbivores." That's about the time our national health got ugly… along with the scenery at the beach.

Since grains don't satisfy hunger for very long, snacking is necessary to stave off cravings. This explains why kids who have been raised as carbivores throw temper tantrums for snacks.

Once snacking becomes habitual, insulin enters the bloodstream full force. Like wind on a fire, blood sugar and insulin begin to inflame belly fat, fatigue and all out laziness. Our internal biochemistry becomes a whirlwind of toxic, fat inflating hormones when we choose low calorie, high-carbohydrate grains. Those are the wrong calories to be counting.

But most people don't see it like this. They accept their fate as a "USDA Approved Carbivore" as a sign of aging and continue their low-fat, high-carb diet. In extreme cases, which have now become far too common, Type II diabetes and cancer set in prematurely.

Without a doubt, calories have inescapable effects on our hormones – the instruments that guide us toward our own unique, healthy perfection. And that's the difference. Calorimeters don't have hormones. Therefore, a calorie count from a calorimeter can't tell you how the body will react to different calories when they are consumed.

The Right Calories Turn You into a HIT Man or Woman

Rather than choosing foods based on low calories, you need to choose foods that provide nutrient-rich calories that promote hormone intelligence. These are calories that come from healthy fats, non-sweet complex carbohydrates, and "complete proteins." Once you learn what each of these are, you can calculate how many of them you need based on your "ideal weight."

It's time to become a calorie snob. From now on, you will only choose the most nutrient-rich calories that get you looking and feeling good via hormone intelligence. These are the calories you will "count" – while ignoring the others. But you do have to make sure you don't get too many. Even too much of the right calories can wreck your physique.

Fat Calories
First and foremost, you're going to reintroduce the fat calorie into your meals. As you learned from Weight Loss Lie #2, eating fat does not make you fat as long as you are selective about the fats you consume and don't overeat.

The calories from healthy fat help to deliver "fat soluble" nutrients such as A, D, E and K throughout the body and help prevent obesity, low energy, lack of concentration and even depression. If any of these conditions are familiar to you, look at how much healthy fat you are consuming.

Healthy fats are essential for good health. They are nutrient rich and don't spike blood sugar and insulin, which is the beginning of hormonal ignorance. In sharp contrast to carbohydrates from grain and sugar, healthy fats tell your body to burn fat and they also make you feel more satisfied. This helps you avoid overeating and becoming psychoglycemic – the state of rage caused by low blood sugar.

Healthy fat calories can be obtained from coconut oil (in tea and coffee or used for cooking), cod-liver oil (this has the omega-3 fats known as EPA and DHA with the added value of naturally occurring vitamin D), olive oil, avocados (omega-9), eggs (raw, scrambled, hard-boiled, whatever), fish, nuts, seeds, pastured pork and poultry and grass-fed beef.

Meals might consist of grass-fed beef (London broil, sausage, New York strip, etc), eggs (the whole egg), pork, beans, rice, chicken, salads, steamed vegetables, coconut oil (for cooking and in tea), fish, small amounts of bread (with REAL butter), cashews, almonds, sunflower seeds, and avocados.

Unhealthy fat calories will make you fat and sick. These include the much talked-about trans fats, the top contributors to obesity and the medical complications that follow. Trans fats disrupt metabolism by invading cell membranes, making them brittle and unresponsive to insulin and glucose, leaving them to float dangerously in the blood. Instead of being renewed by food, cells become resistant to essential nutrients and therefore age quickly.

Trans fats are made in a process is known as "hydrogenation" and are used to increase the shelf life and stability of certain foods. To discover if a food contains trans fat, look at the ingredient list on the food label for the words "shortening," "partially hydrogenated" or "hydrogenated."

If you eat fast food or anything out of a "box" beware! There is a good chance that you are consuming trans fats!

The other fats you need to avoid are those found in vegetable oils such as corn, soy and cottonseed oil (due to high content of carcinogenic omega-6 fatty acids). Healthy replacements for these oils are olive, coconut, avocado and walnut oils (Tables 3 and 4).

Table 3: Fats to Love Summary

Type of Fat	The Skinny	Main Sources
Saturated Fat	Contrary to conventional wisdom, these fats are critical to cellular health, hormone function and metabolism	Grass-fed butter, coconut oil, and the meat and dairy of animals raised on their natural diet (ie. grass-fed cows, pastured poultry, wild game).
Monounsaturated Fat	Critical for smothering inflammation within the body to preserve heart and joint health.	Nuts, avocados and olive oil, walnut and macadamia oils
Omega-3 Fatty Acids	These fats inhibit inflammation and promote fat burning.	Wild Alaskan salmon, sardines, fish oil, cod-liver oil, eggs, grass-fed beef. Plant sources include walnuts, flax seeds and hemp seeds.

Table 4: Fats to Loathe Summary

Type of Fat	The Skinny	Main Sources
Trans Fat	These chemically-manufactured fats do not occur in nature. They cause disease and contribute to obesity. If the words "hydrogenated" or "shortening" are on the list of ingredients, don't eat it.	Processed foods, snack cakes, commercially fried foods, fast food.
Omega-6 Fatty Acids	These fats strongly promote inflammation and are clearly linked to cancer, obesity and heart disease.	Vegetable and seed oils (corn, soybean, cottonseed, peanut, canola, etc.) Read the labels, these are everywhere. This would eliminate commercially fried foods and most processed foods from your diet. Conventionally raised meats (corn-fed cattle, for example) are also much higher in omega-6 fatty acids.

Carbohydrate Calories

The best source of carbohydrate calories are non-sweet, naturally occurring complex carbohydrates from vegetables, especially cruciferous vegetables like broccoli, Brussels sprouts, cabbage, kale, and cauliflower. Regular vegetable consumption curtails weight gain by regulating appetite and ensuring adequate nutrient intake. They're considered low-energy-dense foods, comparing their caloric value to their mass. These carbohydrate calories help prevent overeating and cravings, unlike carbohydrate calories from grains.

They are also rich in cancer fighting compounds known as isothiocyanates, as well as vitamins E, K, A, B-complex and calcium. Calories from green-leafy vegetables also help supply heart healthy CoQ10 in its natural form, unlike what a pill or grain calories would provide. Without the nutrient-rich calories you get from carbohydrates, the energy producing cascade within your body is disabled and fat storage occurs. Energy output is greatly compromised.

Protein Calories

The right protein calories carry the full spectrum of the nine, essential amino acids. Known as "complete proteins," they come from animal sources like grass-fed beef, whey isolate, cottage cheese, and eggs. Since plant based proteins are lacking in essential amino acids, vegetarians and vegans will want to supplement heavy with the complete protein known as brewer's or nutritional yeast.

A lack in protein calories will manifest into poor health and even mental and physical pain very quickly. Your body is always changing. Like a lizard shedding its skin, your skeletal system, muscles and even your internal organs – a phenomenon known as cellular turnover – are replaced in time. This is fueled by nitrogen containing amino acids and proteins. For simplicity, we'll call them "protein calories."

Unlike carbohydrates and fats, protein calories provide the body with the building blocks needed to ensure proper cell turnover as well as the biological production of hormones and peptides that control lean body mass, libido, blood pressure, pain sensitivity, and even our emotions, just to name a few. Without enough protein, your body will decay, fast, rather than live young.

Just as the 26 letters of the alphabet can produce an infinite number of sentences, just twenty amino acids attach and tangle themselves to carve out our physical stature through the biological process known as "turnover." The liver and the pancreas regenerate every year or two (or even quicker if the liver is injured). In the first year of life our entire skeletal system is replaced. And as adults, 10% of it is regenerated annually, unless injury occurs, then it takes place much quicker. The cells that line our gastrointestinal tract, and the epidermis of the skin are exposed to daily challenges, causing them to be replaced every five days and every few weeks, respectively.

Without amino acids from protein calories to push the production of new, healthy tissue, illness and even pain, discomfort and unhappiness prevails. Snap a collarbone flipping over the handlebars of your mountain bike? Ready to go postal because your wife won't get off your ass for loading the dishwasher improperly – or because your hubby can't take the time to do things right? On the edge of beating your boss silly with a coffee mug for micro-managing your every move?

How you feel and react to these pain-stimulating or emotionally-stirring scenarios is partly dictated by your intake of protein, which is not only used to produce the structures of your body, but also your pain-killing hormones.

Just like cell turnover regenerates our physical make-up, our body uses protein to manufacture pain and emotion soothing chemicals in our body known as opioids – on demand. Recently identified as proenkephalin, prodynorphin, and pro-opiomelanocortin, these amino acid conglomerates attenuate life's painful and emotional challenges by working directly on receptors within the brain to smolder fiery sensations.

Powerful enough to sooth even a birthing mother, the complex, three-dimensional design of emotion soothing chemicals is encoded within our genetic map – DNA! Once manufactured in response to our environment, they put pain and emotion on a leash by soothing us as life's trials and tribulations tug on the strings of our Central Nervous System (CNS).

There are still unexplored crevices of knowledge regarding cellular turnover and self-made opiates, but this explains why many people on a high carbohydrate diet – children included – who lack protein calories are typically ill, or reach their "wit's end," and sometimes find life harder to cope with: The innate protection of morphine-like pain killers is dependent on consuming the "right protein calories."

And that's exactly why I designed Whey Advanced. It's the only product in the world that tastes great and has zero sugar, artificial flavors or synthetic hormones. As Mother Nature's miracle food, it provides the body with the full spectrum of the right protien calories for proper hormone intelligence.

In this regard, amino acids represent an entirely new avenue for increasing not only physical health but also mental. Getting the protein calories daily is the first step. **But unlike healthy fats and carbohydrates, your body cannot store proteins to be used later. These calories have to be replenished every day.**

Even if one of the essential amino acids is missing in the diet, turnover will cease, along with the process of producing pain-soothing compounds. Like trying to spell Mississippi without the letter "i," the body is unable to live young and feel emotionally stable.

A missing amino acid or a protein calorie deficiency wreaks biological havoc downstream. It's visible through the appearance of sagging skin, blotchy hair and muscle wasting, all of which water down physical appearance and give rise to a weak, frail look that eventually works against our health, longevity and self-esteem.

Like high blood sugar, this muscle atrophy sets into motion a string of negative, metabolic outcomes like poor energy, osteoporosis and the all-dreadful, belly-fattening insulin resistance, as well as anxiety and depression. The right protein calories are your insurance policy against all of them.

"Healthy foods" that will make you sick and ruin HIT

1. Low Calorie Foods
As adults, most of us have ignored the warning not to eat sugar. We usually pay more attention to how many calories we eat or how many grams of fat we put into our body. This can be a deadly mistake, because most low-calorie and low fat foods are loaded with sugar or "sugar mimics," which raise insulin, just like sugar.

These include sucrose, fructose, glucose, high-fructose corn syrup, monosodium glutamate (MSG), hydrolyzed proteins, hydrogenated oils (trans fat) and milk sugars, such as lactose and maltose. Write these down on your "What Not to Buy at the Grocery Store" list and read the ingredients list on food labels to avoid these fat fertilizers.

2. Soy
Soy was never supposed to be a food. It was cultivated centuries ago in Asia, because dietary sources of protein were scarce and people were starving. In ancient China it was called, "the poor man's cow." Unknowingly, indigenous people reduced many of the anti-nutrients and phytoestrogens (plant-based compounds that mimic the hormone estrogen) via the fermentation process. However, most Americans today eat unfermented soy products, such as soy

milk, soy yogurt, chips, cheese, edamame, tofu, veggie burgers, soy flour in breads and some protein shakes. It is also an ingredient in many "energy" bars and frozen dinners (as hydrolyzed, isolated or concentrated soy protein). In this form, soy protein liberates free amino acids such as glutamate, an excitotoxin that can cause food cravings.

Even if you think you are not eating soy – there is a very good chance you are, unless you know what to look for. Processed foods hide it on the label by calling it other things, like texturized vegetable protein. You should avoid processed foods anyway, but in the rare circumstances where you do eat processed foods, avoid soy products at all costs.

Most soy found in the food supply is genetically modified. But that's not the only reason to avoid this Franken Food. In fact, not even organic varieties of soy are fit for human consumption.

Soy contains "anti-nutrients", including phytates and oxalates, chemicals that interfere with the absorption of important minerals such as zinc and calcium. Other "anti-nutrients" include enzyme inhibitors which interfere with protein digestion and can eventually damage the pancreas.

Soy products also contain compounds which feminize the body and break down muscle. And it is a powerful goitrogen, which means it can significantly slow down the functioning of the thyroid gland.

Soy, and other plants, are poor sources of protein as they are low in certain essential amino acids. Now, consider that soy is the protein source in most baby formulas. In other words, formula-fed babies start out life drinking a cocktail of poor quality protein, powerful estrogen-mimicing compounds and dangerous enzyme inhibitors.

3. Low Fat and No Fat Yogurt
Plain whole milk yogurt (preferably raw and organic), with or without fresh fruit, is delicious, healthy and filling. But this is not what you find in most supermarkets. Most yogurt you see in the grocery store is junk, no matter what health claims are made in the advertisements for these products.

These pasteurized products have very few of the healthy live bacteria cultures remaining. What's more, these heavily sweetened low-fat and fat-free yogurts are not filling and can lead to cravings, overeating, insulin surges and weight gain.

The first problem is that when fat is removed, so is the flavor, texture and satiety value (satiety is the feeling of fullness and satisfaction you feel when there is healthy food in your belly and nutrients in your bloodstream).

To improve the texture, a natural thickener derived from seaweed, called carrageenan, is added. This same ingredient is added to soy, almond, coconut and rice milks, cottage cheese, ice cream and canned pet food. In addition to tumors, carrageenan has been shown to cause inflammation in the gastrointestinal tract. In fact, it is so effective at inducing inflammation, that it is used in lab experiments to do just that.

The second problem is that Big Food promotes a mind-boggling variety of flavors to tempt consumers and keep them hooked, including handy tubes so that kids can conveniently squirt a hit directly into their mouths. Nearly all of these products are sweetened with sugar, fructose, high fructose corn syrup or, perhaps even worse, artificial sweeteners made from toxic chemicals.

Activia's claim to fame is their unique probiotic combo. These friendly bacteria might be beneficial, if they actually make it through the stomach acid alive and if they weren't dumped in a concoction of added fructose, aspartame and carrageenan. Yoplait Light's attraction is that it has, "one third fewer calories than the leading low fat yogurt". Big deal. It also contains both high fructose corn syrup and neurotoxic aspartame!

This is a high-glycemic (even with the aspartame), low-protein disaster, guaranteed to slow your metabolism, lead to cravings, cause weight in the form of fat... and destroy hormone intelligence.

4. Egg Whites

The egg is one of nature's most perfect foods. It is a source of superior protein, great for maintaining and building muscle mass. It is rich in the antioxidants lutein and zeaxanthin that protect the eyes and the arteries, natural forms of vitamins A and D, natural beta-carotene, choline for a healthy nervous system, lots of other vitamins, essential fatty acids, and trace minerals.

And nearly all of this nutritional value is found in the yolk. The egg white is an excellent source of protein, but otherwise, it is a nutritional weakling. Egg white protein is a poor source of the amino acid cysteine, a source of antioxidant sulfur that is abundant in the yolk. And, it takes around six egg whites to make an omelet – what a waste of a perfectly good yolk.

Big Food has capitalized on the misguided belief that yolks are bad, by packaging whites in cartons upon which they stick flawed health claims. Conagra's Egg Beaters Original takes this further by acknowledging that egg whites are missing many nutrients, so they "enrich" their product with synthetic vitamins, minerals, and beta carotene for color. They also add "flavor", although Conagra does not disclose what it is. The added "spices" could be anything, including the excitotoxin MSG and chemical thickeners.

Avoiding foods that stifle HIT, and nourishing your body with those that activate it will equip your "internal pharmacy" with the raw ingredients it needs.

Chapter 5: Meal Planning

Below are a few "HIT Approved" food choices for each meal. Recipes for select dishes can be found on my blog at *www.thepeopleschemist.com/blog*. Simply look for HIT Recipes under "Categories" on the right. Base your food choices on your estimated caloric need and gram ratio of 50% healthy fat, 25% protein, 25% carbohydrate.

It is highly recommended that you purchase *The People's Chemist Approved eating guide* found at *www.myeasydinners.com*. This is the definitive guide for making delicious food that won't harm your hormone intelligence. Written by biochemist, author and chef Kelley Herring, You will receive life-saving information and advice – all of it research-driven and scientifically proven – for making the healthiest meals the entire family loves.

Table 5: Sample Meal Plan

Breakfast Choices	Lunch Choices	Dinner Choices
Organic oatmeal (McCann's Irish Oatmeal) flavored with stevia, real butter, cinnamon,	Egg salad	Pot of Gold
Eggs any style	Chicken salad	Stuffed Beef Peppers, salad
Whey Advanced	Cashews, almonds, walnuts	Big Balls Meat Balls, salad
Organic grapefruit	Organic beef jerky	Salmon dinner with mashed sweet potatoes
Avocado	Cottage cheese	Slow Cooker Latin Chicken
Organic veggie, grass-fed beef omelet	Avocado	Bangers and Mash
Nitrate-free bacon	Vital Choice Tuna Salad	Organic salad with butter lettuce, Cherry tomato, red onion, blue cheese, hard-boiled egg
Organic Sausage	Chicken wrap	Italian salad with mixed greens, banana peppers, red onions, salami, olives, homemade dressing from olive oil, garlic
Brewer's yeast	Canned sardines	Cheese burger night w/ Kosher or grass-fed beef, with sweet potato fries
Greek, full-fat yogurt with blueberries	Chicken sandwich on Ezekial bread	Steaks: T-bone, filet mignon, Petite top sirloin, with Brussels sprouts & bacon

My Easy Dinners

Always know where your food comes from too. You must avoid preservatives, MSG and other pharmafoods, hormones, and environmental toxins that are making their way into our food by the fistful! Two great resources for purchasing real food are *www.uswellnessmeats.com* and *www.vitalchoice.com*

Chapter 6: Workout Less Get More From it

The health and emotional benefits of exercise are profound, but only if you do it right. In fact, by following my HIT exercise principles, you can workout less and get more from it.

Countless studies show that regular exercise dramatically reduces your risk of cancer, heart disease and diabetes, because it forces your internal pharmacy into overdrive (as a result of hormesis, which you've already learned about). It can alleviate chronic pain. It can relieve stress, boost your mood and improve your energy. It can even boost your cognitive ability.

And of course, it not only helps to burn fat and calories, it also sends powerful hormonal signals to your body. That's why it is critical to stay active, because hormonal ignorance sets in after just a few days of being sedentary.

In one study, performed at the University of Missouri-Columbia, researchers allowed a group of rats to voluntarily run on exercise wheels for three weeks. Then they locked the wheels. What they discovered is that within only 48 hours the rats' sensitivity to insulin dropped by one third! And it continued to decrease the longer the rats were inactive.

If you're currently hormonally ignorant and want exercise to work in your favor, then you need to follow the **HIT Exercise Principles** discussed below. Otherwise, the exercise you do will be futile for the purposes of fat loss, no matter how much willpower you take to the gym and how loud you grunt when you're working out.

As a lifetime athlete and chemist studying the effects of physical stress at the molecular level, these principles have been refined over decades to ensure that you spark **hormesis** and so that your body will respond immediately.

Today, actors, elite athletes, MMA fighters, and even soccer moms are using the **HIT Exercise Principles** to get the most out of their exercise routine in the shortest time possible – even as little as 18-minutes.

These principles can be applied to any exercise of your choice including sprinting and gym workouts, as well as programs like Crossfit, P-90X, and others. Or you can simply follow my sample routine below, once you learn and memorize the principles.

The main idea is to focus on the intensity of your exercise, rather than the duration. And as you become accustomed to the activity you're doing, gradually increase the intensity or change the workout.

HIT Exercise Principle #1:
Hit Your Target Heart Rate Every Set

As a pilot, I know my exact heading before I lift off based on where I'm going, obstacles along the way and winds aloft. Otherwise, the chances of arriving safely to my destination decrease. The same is true for exercise. You need to know where you want it to take you, otherwise, you risk not obtaining the desired result.

As a HIT Man or Woman, you need exercise to take your body into thermogenesis – fat burning mode. Like calculating a heading, you need to calculate your "target heart rate" prior to exercise to ensure you trigger this adaptive response.

Your target heart rate is unique to your age and is 60% to 80% of your max heart rate. You can use the simple formula below to decipher your target.

Hitting anything less than your target heart rate is a waste of time because your internal pharmacy will not respond to your efforts. At 37 years old, my target heart beat ranges from 109 beats per minute to 146 BPM. I hit this every set, whether I do 3 or 10, before I stop to rest for my next one. You need to do the exact same. If not, rather than carve out your best body, inferior forms of exercise will simply cause your body to use amino acids and glucose for fuel, which leads to more fat storage and an increase in sugar cravings due to the utilization of blood sugar for fuel.

To determine your target heart rate, you must first determine your maximum heart rate. The formula is: (220 – Your Age) = Your approximate maximum heart rate

Your target heart rate is the range you should hit with every bout of exercise. Your target heart rate is 60% to 80% of your maximum. To measure, count your pulse at the wrist for 15 seconds after your set and multiply that by 4. If you did not hit it, work harder!

Example

Soon to be HIT Man Stan is 45 years old. That means his maximum heart rate is 175.

The formula is (220 – 45) x .60 = 105 bpm. This is the lower end of Stan's target heart rate.

To determine the upper end of his range: (220 – 45) x .80 = 140 bpm.

Therefore the range is 105 to 140 bpm.

Your Target Heart Rate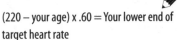

(220 – your age) x .60 = Your lower end of target heart rate

Your lower end of target heart rate =

(220 – your age) x .80 = Your high end of target heart rate

Your high end of target heart rate =

Figure 4. How to determine your target heart rate

HIT Exercise Principle #2: Rest No More than Two Minutes between Sets

Recovery periods are just as important as your sets of exercise. But your periods of rest should not exceed two minutes. Otherwise, instead of activating hormesis leading to hormone intelligence, you'll send a message to your body that the exercise is complete and that it doesn't need to produce the protective hormones for the next set.

When you force your body to recover in just one or two minutes after each set, a surge of protective hormones will flood your central nervous system (CNS), in anticipation of the next "set of destruction."

These are the hormones which are ultimately responsible for anti-aging as well as carving out your best physique. To get them, you must engage in high intensity sets of muscle destruction, followed by set times for rest. Start with two minute rest periods and work toward one. When you can recover in 60 seconds, you'll know that your body is responding to your exercise. Measurable results will be your reward!

HIT Exercise Principle #3:
Don't Consume Sugary Sport Drinks, Bars or Fruit

The optimal time to work out is about 30 minutes after a meal. Do not ingest sports drinks, fruit or anything that tastes sweet after you exercise. Consuming sugar within the first two hours after exercise will cause insulin to surge and shut down your production of human growth hormone (hGH). This occurs as soon as you take your first swig of Vitamin Water and will neutralize your fat loss efforts immediately. In fact, even very small amounts of insulin can decimate your production of growth hormone for eight hours or more.

At the same time, it curbs thermogenesis because insulin and fat burning cannot co-exist! When insulin floats in the blood, it blocks one of the required compounds – Hormone Sensitive Lipase (HSL) – responsible for activating the thermogenic cascade.

Water and tea are the only beverages that won't stifle your hormone intelligence after exercise. My favorite tea is yerba mate for its ability to energize, curb appetite and make you feel great while awaiting your next meal (remember, 5 hours from the last and only 3 per day).

HIT Exercise Principle #4:
Target Large Muscle Groups and Keep them Confused

Your largest muscle groups are going to have the biggest impact on your hormone intelligence. These are the muscles in your legs, butt and back (glutes, quads, hamstrings and lats). The catalyst you need to initiate hormesis is low blood sugar. And since the muscles are the major uptake sites for glucose in the bloodstream, you will see the greatest impact by working the largest muscle groups.

Working your largest muscle groups also triggers the biggest release of growth hormone and testosterone during and after your workout. These two anabolic hormones are vital for burning fat, building muscle and living young.

By alternating your routines and always pushing yourself just past your own personal limits, you keep your muscles guessing and can avoid the plateaus that come with adaptation to exercise. You'll be amazed at what you can do physically and mentally.

So, forget about treadmills, bicep curls and the antiquated bench press. Challenge yourself with full body exercises that test the strength of your largest muscle groups, while simultaneously building the capacity of your heart and lungs.

HIT Exercise Principle #5:
Limit Exercise to 3–5 Times per Week

The surge of hormone intelligence derived from hormesis lasts for days. That means you can continue to derive benefits tomorrow and the day after for the exercise you do today (as long as your intensity is great enough). That also means you don't have to exercise daily.

In fact, without proper rest, you deplete your body of vital nutrients and glycogen. In time, this will cause hormonal ignorance and manifest as accelerated aging. HIT Men and Women can see tremendous benefits from 3–5 workouts per week. It doesn't matter whether you work out two days in a row and then take a day off or if you simply work out every other day.

> ### The Biggest Gains Are Made at Rest
>
> *"The greatest progress occurs when you train hard, then rest deeply."*
>
> Frank Zane
> Fitness Legend

The key is to consistently exercise according to the five **HIT Principles** listed above and don't overdo it. There is nothing wrong with taking a long walk on your days off. In fact, I encourage it. But too much exercise can be even more damaging than too little, so there is no reason to work out at a high intensity more than five days a week.

Sample HIT Exercise Routine

Below are three exercise routines for you to choose from. Each one has three different phases depending on your current level of conditioning – starter, maintenance and extreme. They can be done anywhere with minimal equipment and you only need about 30 minutes from start to finish. Aim to do your routine of choice every other day, spending one to three weeks on each phase then, moving to the next level.

Supplies Needed:

- Jump rope

- Dumbbells

- Exercise mat

- Heart rate monitor (optional)

Warm-up:

- 5-minutes of jump rope or jog

- two sets of 15 push-ups, 25 sit ups, 15 squats or jump squats

- Rest 1–4 minutes

You can use the **HIT Exercise Principles** whenever and wherever you choose and waste no time in the process. Even better, as long as you give it your all, you will know that you are forcing your body into thermogenesis and that you'll be feeling that endorphin high shortly afterwards.

Your best body is absolutely dependent on the proper hormone balance, not excessive exercise. There is no prescription required. You just have to have some guts and determination to activate hormesis by stressing your system in new ways.

This is biochemistry telling us that success lies beyond our comfort zone and that, "Only the smart survive." You'll know the above routine is working by the following measurable results:

- Blood sugar will be lowered to healthy levels after the routine (especially notice-able results can be had by those who are insulin resistant or Type II diabetic)

- Recovery times will shorten between your sets

- Dumbbell weight will increase

- Resting heart rate will drop (It is best to measure your resting heart rate in the morning just after you wake up and before you have any coffee)

- Friends and family will notice your leaner, healthier physique

Table 6: HIT Routine 1 – Starter phase

Exercise	Duration	Recovery	Sets
Air Squats	1 minute	2 minutes	2
Squats or Jump squats with dumbbell curl to press	1 minute	2 minutes	2
Beginner burpees	1 minute	2 minutes	2

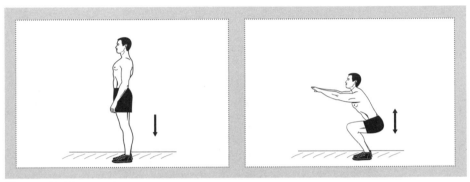

Figure 5. Air squats

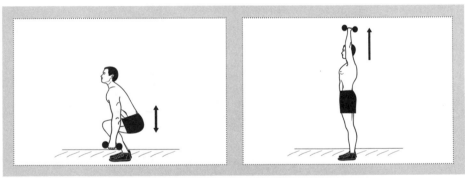

Figure 6. Squats or Jump squats with dumbbell curl to press

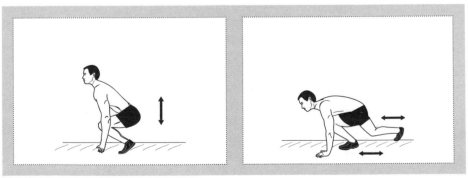

Figure 7. Beginner burpees

Table 7: HIT Routine 1 – Maintenance phase

Exercise	Duration	Recovery	Sets
Standing jump squats (use dumbbells if needed)	2 minutes	1 minute	2
Weighted lunges	2 minutes	1 minute	2
Burpees	2 minutes	1 minute	3

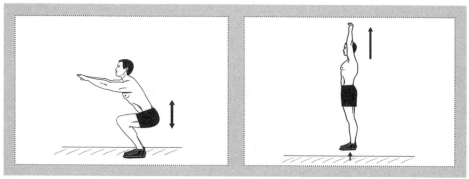

Figure 8. Standing jump squats (use dumbbells if needed)

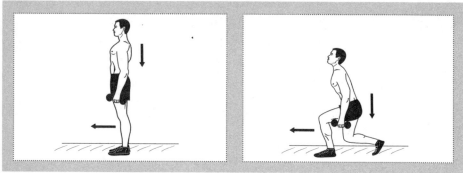

Figure 9. Weighted lunges

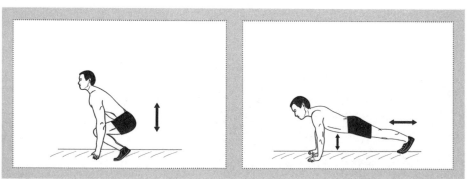

Figure 10. Burpees

Table 8: HIT Routine 1 – Extreme phase

Exercise	Duration	Recovery	Sets
Squats or Jump squats with dumbbell curl to press	2 minutes	1 minute	2
Lunges with dumbbell curl to military press	2 minutes	1 minute	2
Burpees with dumbbell curl to press	2 minutes	1 minute	3

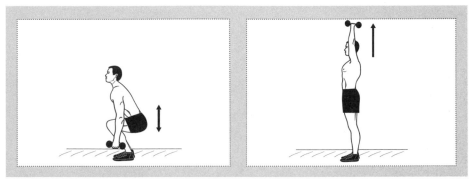

Figure 11. Squats or Jump squats with dumbbell curl to press

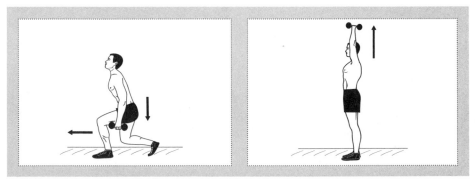

Figure 12. Lunges with dumbbell curl to military press

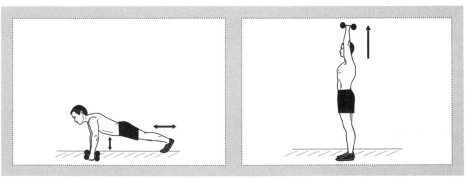

Figure 13. Burpees with dumbbell curl to press

Table 9: HIT Routine 2 – Starter phase

Exercise	Duration	Recovery	Sets
Thrusters with light dumbbells	1 minute	2 minutes	2
Sit-ups	1 minute	2 minutes	2
Walking lunge with light dumbbells	1 minute	2 minutes	2

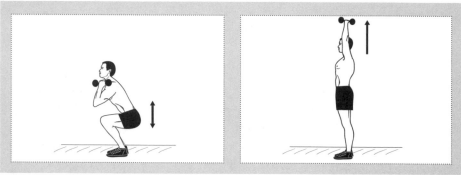

Figure 14. Thrusters with light dumbbells

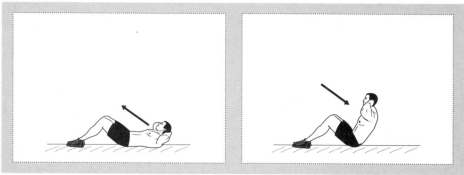

Figure 15. Sit-ups

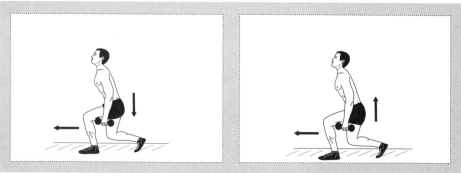

Figure 16. Walking lunge with light dumbbells

Table 10: HIT Routine 2 – Maintenance phase

Exercise	Duration	Recovery	Sets
Thrusters with light dumbbells	2 minutes	1 minute	2
Sit-ups	2 minutes	1 minute	2
Walking lunge with light dumbbells	2 minutes	1 minute	3

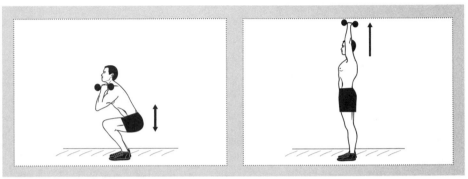

Figure 17. Thrusters with light dumbbells

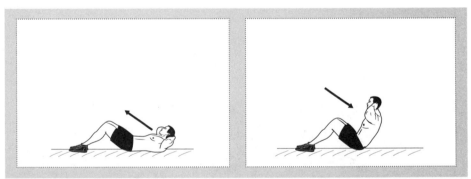

Figure 18. Sit-ups

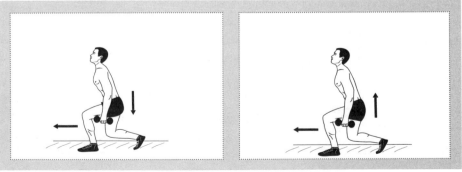

Figure 19. Walking lunge with light dumbbells

Table 11: HIT Routine 2 – extreme phase

Exercise	Duration	Recovery	Sets
Thrusters with dumbbells	2 minutes	1 minute	2
Weighted Sit-ups	2 minutes	1 minute	2
Walking lunge with dumbbell over head	2 minutes	1 minute	3

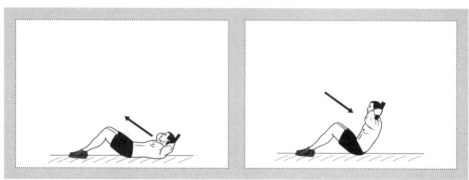

Figure 20. Thrusters with dumbbells

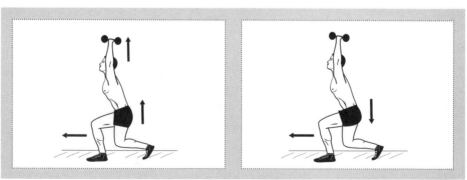

Figure 21. Weighted Sit-ups

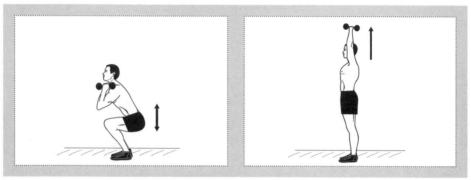

Figure 22. Walking lunge with dumbbell over head

Table 12: HIT Routine 3 – Starter phase

Exercise	Duration	Recovery	Sets
Air squats	1 minute	2 minutes	2
Thrusters with dumbbells	1 minute	2 minutes	2
Man makers	1 minute	2 minutes	2

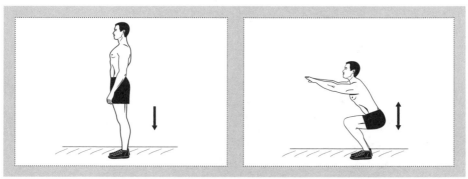

Figure 23. Air squats

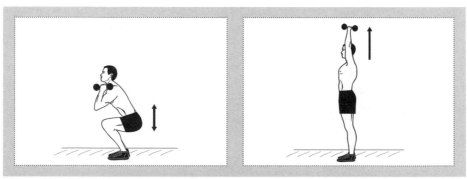

Figure 24. Thrusters with dumbbells

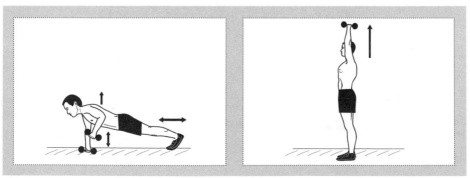

Figure 25. Man makers

Table 13: HIT Routine 3 – Maintenance phase

Exercise	Duration	Recovery	Sets
Air squats	2 minutes	1 minute	2
Thrusters with dumbbells	2 minutes	1 minute	2
Man makers	2 minutes	1 minute	3

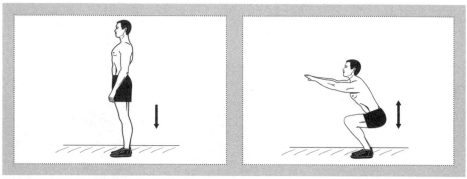

Figure 26. Air squats

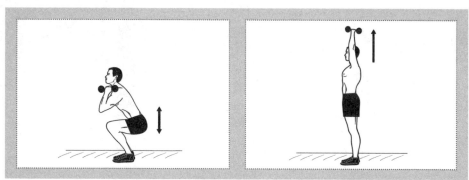

Figure 27. Thrusters with dumbbells

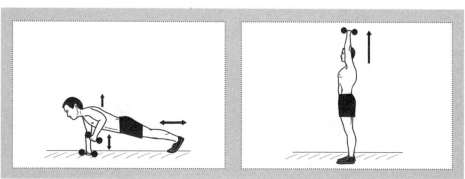

Figure 28. Man makers

Table 14: HIT Routine 3 – Extreme phase

Exercise	Duration	Recovery	Sets
Squats to curl and press	2 minutes	1 minute	2
Thrusters with dumbbells	2 minutes	1 minute	2
Man makers	2 minutes	1 minute	3

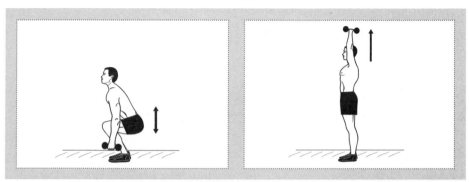

Figure 29. Squats to curl and press

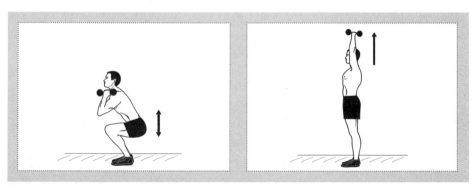

Figure 30. Thrusters with dumbbells

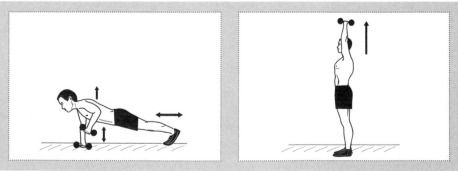

Figure 31. Man makers

Chapter 7: Better than Steroids – Hormone Intelligence Therapy Boosters

Just like a meth lab needs cough syrup as the starting material for its final product, the body has requirements for its internal pharmacy. In my book, *Over-The-Counter Natural Cures*, I taught that we must give key nutrients from nature so that it can become our biggest ally in healing. And as you've learned so far, this is also true if we want to become a HIT Man or HIT Woman.

To increase, or "potentiate," the effect of HIT, nature has provided key ingredients that help both men and women. Unlike Hormone Replacement Therapy (HRT) or the use of bioidentical hormones, natural "hormone boosters" will not "bioaccumulate" or artificially throw your own hormones out of whack. They simply help optimize your unique hormone output, balance and sensitivity.

These are not mandatory. And should only be used once men have less than 15% body fat and women 20%. When used properly, in the right dose and in combination, they can provide athletes with enhanced hormone intelligence. The best way to begin using them is to start with sarsaparilla, daily. Once you are comfortable with its use, you can introduce a combo of all four once every three to five days. Beware of minor side effects such as low blood sugar and agitation. If they set in, reduce the dose or take some time off (Table 15).

Table 15: Hormone Intelligence Therapy Boosters

Potentiator	Mechanism	Starting Dose	Best Brand
Sarsaparilla	Optimizes testosterone / estrogen balance and sensitivity among men and women. Great for increasing strength, shortening recovery times, boosting immunity as a natural antibiotic and antiviral. Also works to diminish acne	500 to 1,500 mg daily per 150lbs of body weight	Nature's Herbs Sarsaparilla from www.vitacost.com
Fenugreek	Increases testosterone and DHT (strength producing hormone) levels and sensitivity	500 to 1,000 mg daily per 150 lbs of body weight	Testofen Fenugreek by Swanson at Amazon.com
Eurycoma Longifolia	Reduce estrogen, optimize estrogen / testosterone balance, increase free testosterone and sensitivity, increases sperm count preventing male infertility	100 to 400 mg daily per 100 lbs of body weight	Swanson Passion Products from Amazon.com
Stinging Nettle	Reduces estrogen by lowering aromatase enzyme, which converts testosterone to estrogen	300 to 500mg daily per 150lbs of body weight	Eclectic Institute at www.vitacost.com

Chapter 8: Secrets to Raising HIT

Get Plenty of Sunshine

Exposing as much of your body as possible to sunlight for 20–45 minutes three to five times per week elicits the biological production of vitamin D and a neuropeptide known as Melanocyte Stimulating Hormone (MSH). Together, these compounds prevent fat storage, control appetite and normalize insulin and blood glucose levels. Increased thermogenesis is also a result.

Without exposure to sunshine, excess fat storage occurs and the body screams for carbohydrates and sweets.

Note: The benefits of sun exposure are not attained if sunscreen is used. Most sunscreens actually contribute to skin damage (i.e. cancer) and prevent it from responding in a healthy manner to sunshine as outlined in *Over-The-Counter Natural Cures*. Fortunately, exposing your skin to 20 to 45 minutes of sunshine does not mandate the need for sun block. If you live in cold climates, pray that summer arrives as soon as possible, and as you're waiting, supplement with Carlson's Norwegian Cod Liver Oil.

Drink Lemon Water Between Meals

The acid – a compound known as limonene – from lemon slows stomach emptying and digestion. Consuming a full squeezed lemon in 20 ounces of purified water with a meal can lower blood sugar as much as 30%. By controlling blood sugar, the body can better rebound from the post meal insulin spike and begin burning fat sooner instead of storing it.

Consume Psyllium Husk

Like acid from lemons, the fiber known as psyllium husk also slows stomach emptying and digestion. Consuming a teaspoon in water before a meal once to twice per week will prevent a spike in insulin and blood sugar over time. Post meal fat burning will begin much sooner by using psyllium husk.

Limit Alcohol Consumption

While the effects are not nearly as pronounced as sugar, the excess consumption of alcohol can disrupt your hormone intelligence. In particular, alcohol causes testosterone and human growth hormone to drop, while estrogen rises. Over time, this can exacerbate insulin resistance.

If you do drink alcohol, limit your consumption to sulfite-free, organic wine. I believe the healthiest wines to indulge are those made by California winery, Orleans Hill. Their two most popular are, Our Daily Red (which you can find at Whole Foods) or Well Read (carried by Trader Joe's). These wines have no added sugar or sulfites and can be enjoyed without worrying about what toxic additives have been tossed in by the manufacturer. (See the PC TV interview with the wine maker at www.thepeopleschemist.com)

Avoid mixers that contain sugar and artificial ingredients. Stick to soda water, or a sparkling beverage like Zevia (www.zevia.com) for cocktails.

To further lessen the negative effects of alcohol, consume it with a meal consisting of protein and fat. This will slow its absorption into the bloodstream and prevent the negative impact on weight gain due to insulin and blood glucose levels.

Avoid Prescription Drugs that Cause Obesity

Commonly used prescription drugs can disrupt your metabolism. When used long term (6 months or more), these drugs commonly cause obesity and will negate the benefits of HIT.

The detrimental hormonal and metabolic effects of these drugs cannot even be overcome with rigorous workouts and a regimented diet. I have seen the effects of "drug-induced obesity" hundreds of times over the years in readers who have written to me and clients I have consulted with on a personal basis. The most common obesity-inducing drugs are those used for birth control, high blood pressure (beta blockers such as Atenolol), depression (SSRIs), and type II diabetes (sulfonylureas such as Amaryl and thiazolidinediones such as Avandia).

Most drugs have natural alternatives that work better and safer, for about $10 per month! To learn more, read my book *Over-The-Counter Natural Cures* (available anywhere books are sold) to discover where to obtain them and how to apply them to your HIT goals!

Chapter 9: What Your Best Body Really Is

Your "best body" is not the contrived, air-brushed images of Hollywood. Nor is it the roided-out, puffy look popularized by bodybuilding. It's your own unique physique based on a perfect balance of fat and muscle. To aim for it, start monitoring your body fat percentage as you get near your "ideal weight." Men should aim for 11% – 14% body fat, women 15% – 19%.

Additionally, you can calculate how much muscle you pack on as a HIT Man or Woman using "lean body mass" comparisons. Lean body mass is the weight of your bones, water, glycogen, skin, hair, organs and muscle – everything except

Example

For example, at 205 pounds and 30% body fat, my lean body mass was 143.5 lbs. (205 – 61.5).

Your lean body mass

Your lean body mass = (Current weight) – (Total pounds of fat) =

Figure 32. How to calculate lean body mass

fat. To obtain lean body mass, get your body fat parentage calculated then subtract your total pounds of fat from your body weight.

Now, here's the fun part. Over time, calculate how much muscle you have put on (or lost) by subtracting your starting lean body mass from your current lean body mass.

Example

For example, my starting lean body mass was 143.5 pounds. After reaching 175 pounds, my body fat percentage was 11%. Therefore, my new lean body mass was 156 pounds. Subtracting my previous lean mass of 143.5, showed that I gained 12.5 pounds of muscle (156 − 143.5). That was over a 90-day period.

Your starting lean body mass

Your starting lean body mass:

Your current lean body mass:

Muscle gained = (Current lean body mass) − (Starting lean body mass) =

Figure 33. How to calculate muscle gained

Don't let excuses get in your way!

You're only six habits away from your best body – and about 90 days. Just remember that all the habits go together. Like four wheels on a car, removing one habit from the plan will put a stop to forward progress. So, here's a look at all the habits together.

1. If it tastes sweet, spit it out

2. Make purified water your drink of choice

3. Restrict calories for HIT, not starvation

4. Use thermogenic aids

5. Sleep like a drunken bum naturally

6. Exercise to activate hormesis

With these, you can now choose your own hormonal fate, regardless of any previous excuses – even the "it's in my genes," excuse. Genetics are simply the bullet in the gun. Your habits pull the trigger. A lot of people don't want to acknowledge this, but studies from the Human Genome project prove it – you were not meant to live overweight. Your genes respond to your habits, not the other way around. We might not all look the same, but we all can all avoid poor health that stems from weight gain...Sure there are exceptions, but exceptions don't make the rule.

There will be slip-ups. Slip-ups are okay. What matters most is that if you do slip-up you don't stay down. Whether it's a period of poor eating, lack of exercise or even an injury, as a HIT Man or Woman, you'll have the hormones that will enable you to get back up.

As sure as a bowling ball will knock down pins, your hormones will react to the HIT breakthrough. And as you know by now, it won't take hardcore willpower. The key nutrition, supplement and lifestyle habits that govern Hormone Intelligence Therapy were founded on SIMPLICITY.

The pursuit of your best body should enrich your life, not detract from it. That's why there are only six simple habits to live by. Do them consistently and you can look forward to tightly defined muscles, the capacity to outperform your peers by a tremendous margin and if you're really determined, having abs or a back side that people will look twice at. But best of all, that 6 foot strand of code that dictates your hormone intelligence (or ignorance), DNA, will forever be protected and guide you toward perfect health and slow the hands of time – without fad diets and prescription drugs, and ever prevent you from eating too fucking much.

Glossary

acesulfame K K, for potassium. An artificial sweetener known as Sunett or Sweet One. It exacerbates feelings of low blood sugar.

adenosine Ado; an inhibitory neurotransmitter that promotes sleep and suppresses arousal. It is blocked by caffeine. The chemical name refers to a sugar molecule secreted by the glands.

adiponectin A protein hormone involved in regulating glucose levels as well as fatty acid breakdown. It comes from a combination of Latin and Greek words that mean, "protein that has an effect on fat."

adipocytes Literally, fat cells.

agonist A chemical substance capable of activating a receptor to induce a response.

amaranth Seeds used as a cereal grain.

Amphetamines Speed; they curb hunger by decreasing the appetite. Some people abuse this class of drugs in order to lose weight; others, to be able to get around Manhattan on any weekday.

amylin Hormone secreted by the pancreas along with insulin. It plays a role in glycemic control.

anabolic Describing a process by which food is changed into living tissue; also referring to constructive metabolism.

antineoplastons A peptide that destroys, inhibits or prevents new cellular growths from spreading. These give cancer the smack-down before it knows what hit it.

aromatase Enzyme responsible for converting testosterone to estrogen. If you're taking a lot of testosterone, while still insulin resistant, you probably have a nice set of hooters yourself now. Those are not pecs - they're "moobs."

aspartame A very sweet artificial neurotoxin made in a lab. As it breaks down in the body, one of its byproducts is formaldehyde - the same stuff they keep the frogs immersed in, in high school biology classes.

ATP Adenosine Tri-Phosphate, the energizing molecule formed by the body. ATP transports chemical energy within the cells for metabolism. As blood sugar rises, ATP production decreases along with energy and libido.

beta blocker A drug that prevents stimulation of increased cardiac action, used to treat angina and reduce high blood pressure. Essentially, the metabolic switches that set fat metabolism into motion, beta-receptors, are blocked. The result is fat storage and muscle wasting despite diet and exercise, due to the introduction of a beta blocker.

BMR Basal Metabolic Rate. The rate at which the body uses energy while at rest to keep vital functions going.

Bowman-Birk Inhibitor A protein enzyme inhibitor found in soybeans.

Calcitonin An amino acid hormone that helps regulate calcium levels and inhibits the loss of calcium from bone to the blood.

capsaicin The active component contained in chili peppers.

catacholamines Fight-or-flight hormones produced by the adrenal glands in response to stress. They are part of the sympathetic nervous system. Catacholamines present in the human body include epinephrine, norepinephrin and dopamine, which act as natural stimulants in response to stress.

CCK Cholecystokinin, as in CholeCystoKinin. See **cholecystokinin**.

cholecystokinin A hormone secreted by the upper portion of the intestine that stimulates contraction of the gall bladder and increases secretion of the pancreatic juices, which then helps the body break down food into a form that can be used for energy. The word comes from a combination of Greek words that mean, "hormone that moves the gall bladder."

Citrus Aurantium Bitter orange. A spiny evergreen tree that bears fruit which is used as a stimulant and appetite suppressant. Slivers of the rind are also used to make marmalade.

Clenbuterol Synthetic steroids used to treat asthma. It is abused by body builders to induce thermogenesis and make them look more massive, like "The Governator", but it can cause nerve damage, nervousness and heart problems.

cytokines A large and diverse family of protein molecules secreted by the nervous system and immune systems. From the Greek *cyto-* cell + *-kinos* movement.

DHA An omega-3 fatty acid, which is an unsaturated fatty acid found in cod liver oil. The initials come from the chemical word, DocosaHexaenoic Acid, derived from Greek, which describes its content: do, from duo, "two" + shortened form of eicosa, "twenty" (there are 22 carbon atoms in the molecule) + hexa, "six" (number of unsaturated bonds) + -ene, denoting a compound + -oic, the form of.

DHEA The main steroidal hormone of the adrenals, gonads and brain. It is the most abundant circulating hormone in humans. DHEA converts to other hormones, including estrogen and testosterone. It plays a role in strength, memory, fertility, memory, cardiovascular health, memory and longevity (just making sure you're still paying attention). An inferior form of DHEA may also be synthesized in the lab and used in "bioidentical" drug design. The abbreviation comes from the letters of a biochemical compound that indicates it's structure and where it comes from in the body – hydrogen and oxygen, secreted mainly by the adrenals.

DHT DiHydroTestosterone. A male sex and strength producing hormone.

einkorn A wild species of wheat. The name comes from a German word for "single grain."

emmer A variety of wheat, also called faro in Italy. It was one of the first crops domesticated in the ancient world.

EPA An omega-3 fatty acid, which is an unsaturated fatty acid found in cod liver oil. The initials come from the chemical word, EicosaPentaenoic Acid, derived from Greek, which describes its content: eicosa, "twenty" (the number of carbon atoms in the molecule) + penta, "five" (the number of unsaturated bonds) + -ene, denotes a compound + -oic, the form of.

Ephedra A Chinese herbal remedy for asthma and hay fever as well as the common cold. In Chinese, ma huang, constricts blood vessels and increases blood pressure and heart rate. Ephedra-containing dietary supplements have been linked to a high rate of side effects and a number of deaths, therefore the FDA banned its use on April 12, 2004. No TPC products contain ephedra at all.

EPO ErythroPOietin is a hormone that controls red blood cell production by acting on precursors in the bone marrow.

estradiol The most potent and dominant female sex hormone. It is produced by the human body from puberty to menopause and is the dominant circulating hormone during pregnancy. It is involved in over 400 functions of the female body. An inferior molecular form of estradiol may also be synthesized in the lab and combined with synthesized estrone, estriol and progesterone, to make a "bioidentical." Funny enough, the word comes from Greek, which loosely translates into "hormone that is twice as annoying as usual."

estriol The weakest estrogen, mainly produced by the placenta during pregnancy and not otherwise measurable. An inferior molecular form of estriol may be synthesized in a lab and combined with the other franken-hormones to make a "bioidentical." The word comes from Greek and loosely translates as the "hormone that makes a woman three times as mad." Sounds like the Greeks knew what they were talking about.

estrone This is the estrogen left after menopause, made primarily by body fat. An inferior molecular form of estrone may also be synthesized in the lab and combined with other forms to make a "bioidentical." The word comes from Greek and loosely translates as the "hormone that drives a women mad."

excitotoxin A substance, such as glutamate, that damages and kills nerve cells.

faro See **emmer**.

fat soluble vs water soluble Vitamins are classified as either fat soluble (vitamins A, D, E and K) or water soluble (vitamins B and C). This difference determines how each vitamin acts within the body. "Soluble" means, that can be dissolved or capable of passing into solution, therefore, some vitamins are not capable of being dissolved in water, but can be dissolved in lipids (fat). Fat soluble vitamins are usually absorbed by fats and travel into the general blood circulation within the body, where they are then stored in body tissues. Once they are stored, they tend to remain there, so if a person takes too much of a fat soluble vitamin, over time they can have too much of that vitamin present in their body. A deficiency in fat soluble vitamins can be created if a person's fat intake is too low. Water soluble vitamins are capable of being dissolved in water and therefore simply require water. Dehydration could contribute to a deficiency of water soluble vitamins.

frankenfood "Food" made in a lab. Think Frankenstein.

Garcinia Cambogia A plant native to Indonesia, commonly known as Gambooge. Its fruit is yellowish and pumpkin-shaped. In traditional Indian medicine, it is used for bowel complaints, edema, delayed menstruation, constipation and intestinal parasites. In weight loss products it is used as an appetite suppressant and for energy.

glucagon A hormone produced in the pancreas, which raises blood glucose levels. Its effect is opposite that of insulin, which lowers blood glucose levels. It is derived from the Greek *gleukos*, sweetness plus *-on*, denoting a hormone.

glycemic How carbohydrates in food effect blood sugar levels. High glycemic foods have an increased effect on blood sugar levels. Low glycemic foods have a lessened effect.

gluconeogenesis Glucose formation from proteins or fats.

glycogen A substance produced by the liver and muscles, which is changed into a simple sugar as the body needs it.

ghrelin A hormone produced by cells lining the upper portion of the stomach that stimulate hunger. [< g(rowth) h(ormone)-rel(easing peptide) + suf. -in, used to indicate hormone]

goitrogen A substance that affects the thyroid gland and may cause a swelling in the front of the neck.

hormesis A biological effect in which a toxic substance acts like a stimulant in small doses, but is an inhibitor in large doses. The idea is that a little bit of stress (toward improving one's health and stress tolerance) prepares the body to deal with larger stresses. Therefore, exercising to activate hormesis is moderate exercise in order to activate the body's own pharmacy in the form of healthy hormone response. It is derived from Greek, meaning "set in motion."

hydroxycitric acid (HCA) A derivative of citric acid found in a variety of tropical plants, which regulates lipid metabolism.

hyperinsulinemia Excess levels of insulin circulating in the blood than expected relative to the level of glucose. It is usually associated with type II diabetes, but it can also result from a variety of metabolic conditions.

IGF-1 Insulin-like Growth Factor.

interleukin (IL-6) Originally, proteins that act as a means of communication by and on white blood cells. The immune system depends on white blood cells. The IL-6 series induces inflammation as a reactive response.

isothiocyanate A nitrogen-carbon-sulfur compound that combines easily with other compounds. They are cancer-fighting compounds contained in non-sweet, complex carbohydrate vegetables. The word means "equal parts of sulfur, nitrogen and carbon" in Greek - hence the phrase, "It's all Greek to me" was probably first spoken by an organic chemist. Too bad Americans were not the first people to civilize the ancient world. All these terms would be so much easier to understand.

Kamut® Product name for an ancient grain closely related to durum wheat.

ketones Substances that are made when the body breaks down fat for energy.

leptin A hormone that plays a key role in regulating energy intake and expenditure, including appetite and metabolism. [<Gr leptos, thin]

macrophage chemoattractant protein (MCP-1) When a white blood cell enters damaged tissue through the interior layer of a blood vessel it undergoes a series of changes that results in a macrophage. Macrophage comes from a Greek word meaning, "big eater." White blood cells in general are attracted to damaged tissue due to a biochemical cascade of damaged cells, pathogens and other stimuli released by these new forms of white blood cells, which in turn attracts more simple white blood cells to the area. Macrophages engulf (or eat) pathogens and can survive up to several months. They protect the body by ingesting harmful particles, bacteria and dead or dying cells. The rush of all this aid to a local area of inflammation can cause even more inflammation and bring about an even more dangerous situation in a body that already has restricted blood flow due to poor cardiovascular health. Imagine a car accident on a major freeway – already in need of repair – during rush hour. Now imagine 20 fire trucks, 30 ambulances, 40 paramedics and 50 police cars all rushing to the scene. What do you think is going to happen to all the traffic? How long is it going to take all that "aid" to clear out after they're satisfied they've filled out all the paperwork and done their job? That gives you some idea of what happens when the immune system goes into overdrive in a body that is already unhealthy.

Melanocyte A pigment in the skin responsible for color. It comes from a Greek word for "black."

Meridia A fat loss drug used as an appetite suppressant, but it can also cause back pain, constipation, dizziness, dry mouth, flu symptoms and headaches.

Neotame Artificial sweetener made by Nutrasweet that's about 10,000 times sweeter than sucrose. It's far from "tame."

neovascularisation The growth of new blood vessels.

neuropeptides Any of various short-chain amino-acid compounds, as endorphins, that function as hormones in the endocrine system and influence the function of the nerve cells in the nervous system.

Omega-9 A family of unsaturated fatty acids which have in common a carbon-carbon double bond in the 9th position. It is not considered essential, because the human body can create it from Omega-3 fats. It is found in olive oil and avocados. See **Saturated vs unsaturated fats**.

Omega-6 A family of unsaturated fatty acids that have in common a carbon-carbon double bond in the 6th position. It is found in most vegetable oils and has been linked to an increase in breast cancer in women and prostate cancer in men. See **Saturated vs unsaturated fats**.

Omega-3 Fats These are considered the essential fatty acids. They are necessary for human health, but the body cannot make them on its own. You have to get them through food, such as, fish (salmon, tuna, halibut & other seafood, including algae), some plants and nut oils. See **Saturated vs unsaturated fats**.

oxalates A substance found in soy, spinach, rhubarb and other vegetables and nuts that interferes with the body's absorption of calcium.

peptides A compound formed of 2 or more amino acids linked together, which occurs during digestion.

PGC1-Alpha A complex term for a co-activator that regulates the genes involved in energy metabolism. You only need to know what the acronym means if you are studying organic chemistry (otherwise, it's just not important).

Phentermine A drug used to speed weight loss by decreasing appetite.

phenylalanine An essential amino acid contained in protein. It's "essential", because your body cannot produce it; it needs to be eaten.

phenylalkylketones Organic alkaloid compounds found in ginger root responsible for improved circulation and preventing motion sickness.

phosphorylation A process in organic chemistry, that introduces a phosphate group into an organic molecule or protein. In this case, the phosphorylation of sugars allows the cells of the muscles to accumulate "high energy" molecules that can be expended during exercise as long as the glucose vacuums are not "gummed-up" with excess insulin.

phytates A substance found in plants, especially soy and cereal grains that interferes with the absorption of calcium, zinc, iron and other nutrients.

phytoestrogen A plant derived estrogen, such as soy and soy products.

prodynorphin A hormone formed from multiple amino acid compounds that has a sedative effect on the body. It is involved in how the cells communicate and send energy messages throughout the body, with the effect of attenuating pain.

proenkephalin A protein conglomerate formed in the brain and adrenals that is a precursor for several neuropeptides.

progesterone A steroid hormone that prepares the uterus for the fertilized ovum and the mammary glands for milk secretion. It is derived by the body from precursors that are themselves derived from cholesterol. It is relatively low in children and postmenopausal women. An inferior molecular form of progesterone may be synthesized in the lab, which is then combined with other synthesized estrogens in "bioidentical" drug design. It comes from Latin and means "hormone that comes before carrying (a baby)."

pro-opiomelanocortin A residue inactive precursor from which a hormone is derived, found in the pituitary gland.

prostaglandin Lipid compounds derived from fatty acids. Originally, it was thought to be secreted by the prostate gland, but later found to originate all over the body.

psycho-glycemic A state of rage caused by low blood sugar.

PYY Peptide YY. This hormone is released in the lower small intestine and colon. It decreases hunger, by acting like a brake, causing a feeling satiety. Its name comes from Peptide tYrosine tYrosine.

resistin A relatively newly discovered protein that has been observed to be involved in insulin resistance and obesity, which is also linked to inflammation activity.

Saturated vs unsaturated fats Fats contain long hydrocarbon chains. The type of fat determines its character and how healthy it is. Saturated fats are evenly filled out with hydrogen and remain solid at room temperature, such as, butter, dairy products and the white layer in a cut of meat. Double bonds in the hydrocarbon chain results in an unsaturated fat. A single double bond is called a monounsaturated fat. Multiple double bonds are called polyunsaturated fats. There are three families of polyunsaturated fats worth paying attention to: Omega-3, Omega-6 & Omega-9. To keep it simple, you need to eat foods that contain natural Omega-3, because your body cannot manufacture them, therefore they're essential. Your body can make Omega-9 fats from Omega-3. You should avoid Omega-6 fats found in vegetable oils.

sida cordifolia Country mallow. A shrub native to India. The heart-shaped leaf is referred to as cordifolia. In Ayurvedic medicine the herb is used as an anti-inflammatory of the mucous membranes, for treating cancer and encouraging liver regrowth. It also has stimulant properties affecting the CNS and heart.

spelt A type of wheat that was common in Europe during the Middle Ages, now newly marketed as a health food.

SSRI An acronym for Sure-fire Source of Repeat Income for the pharmaceutical industry. They would rather you believe it stands for Selective Serotonin Re-uptake Inhibitor. However, they have no test to prove its need nor any blood test to prove that this process occurs. One thing it will definitely do is block hormone intelligence.

Sucralose (Splenda) An artificial sweetener that contains chlorine and is 600 times sweeter than sugar. It's made in a lab, therefore it doesn't belong in your body.

sulfonylurea An antidiabetic consisting of several drugs that reduce the level of glucose in the blood.

sympathetic nervous system (SNS) The part of the nervous system that has to do with the involuntary responses of the body to alarm, such as speeding up the heart rate and the enlargement of the pupils.

telomeres A region at the ends of our DNA, which protects the ends of our chromosomes from deterioration and fusion with neighboring chromosomes. Think of them as the plastic ends of a shoelace for comparison. The word comes from Greek for "end-part."

Testosterone Male sex hormone. This is the "My House, My Rules, My Way or the Highway" hormone. Some women are a little too dominant in this one, the same way some men who have too much estrogen, are reaching for their tissues, while watching the Lifetime channel.

thiazolidinedione A class of drugs that target insulin resistance (type II diabetes).

triiodothyronine (T3) A hormone secreted by the thyroid gland that affects almost every physiological function in the body, such as growth, development, metabolism, body temperature and heart rate.

tumor necrosis factor-a (TNF-a) A biochemical factor that regulates the immune cells and plays a part in the response to local inflammation along with a host of other factors. TNF-a is a protein molecule that aids intercellular communication. It is produced by the nervous system in response to inflammation, in order to induce apoptosis (cell suicide) so as to prevent growth of rogue cells (tumors).

Wellbutrin An antidepressant drug also marketed for weight loss, which just happens to be one of its many side effects. Unfortunately, anti-depression is not one of its effects. It can also cause uncontrollable shaking of a part of the body (turn that music up – I got a dance in me that needs to come out!), drowsiness, dizziness, vomiting, headache and constipation, among others. Oh yeah, I'm dizzy and tired, I'm throwing up, I can't stop shaking, I have a headache and I'm constipated – Yeah, I feel much better!

vitamin K Vitamin K is a fat soluble vitamin, so your body stores it in fat tissue and the liver. It is best known for its role in helping blood clot, or coagulate, properly. It also plays an important role in bone health. The "K" comes from its German name, Koagulationsvitamin.

Xenical A drug used to help people lose weight. Some of its side effects include bowel movement urgency (just how urgent?), gas with discharge, inability to control bowel movements (ok, that's pretty urgent) and increased number of bowel movements – wow! What's the upside again?

zeaxanthin A carotenoid that helps protect eye health. It comes from a Greek word for "yellow substance."

Notes and Calculations